# "We highly recommend this book!"

Howard and Jeanne Hendricks

"No couple in America is better qualified to write a book on this topic than Bill and Vonette Bright. They have written a classic that will impact thousands of American families for years to come."

**Pat and Jill Williams**
Co-authors, *Rekindled*

"It is refreshing indeed to have a couple like Bill and Vonette Bright, who have been so active in Christian ministry, share their marital experiences with others . . . and to know that here is a couple who continue to manifest a godly lifestyle and a warm, loving relationship—after 40 years of marriage!"

**David and Carole Hocking**
Co-authors, *Romantic Lovers* and
*Good Marriages Take Time*

"Bill and Vonette's untiring enthusiasm in the Lord's service has always been an inspiration to my husband and me. And we value their love and friendship over the years."

**Ruth Graham**

"Bill and Vonette will long be remembered as godly role models with a glowing love relationship with each other. They have been a living example of the Spirit-filled life in handling stress in the ministry, separation because of excessive travel, and success as a result of God's blessing."

**Tim and Beverly LaHaye**
Authors, Speakers

"When a marriage thrives in the midst of levels of life stress that engineers would claim is structurally impossible to withstand, we all want to know the secret. There are no hairline cracks in this marriage. Bill and Vonette Bright love each other in a manner that not even their fast pace as two world travelers can shake. We highly recommend this book, written by two close friends and role models, as a time-proven solution to one of the biggest threats to today's marriages."

**Howard and Jeanne Hendricks**
Chairman, Center for Christian Leadership
Distinguished Professor, Dallas Theological Seminary


"*Managing Stress in Marriage* is undoubtedly one of the most exciting and spiritually stimulating books on a delicate subject. It's mandatory reading for every Christian worker as well as laypeople. I predict it will be a bestseller."

**Jack Van Impe**


"A candid peek into the lives of two effective and faithful Christian leaders who made their ministry and marriage work. In these pages you will not find an aloof relationship which you're unable to relate to, but an honest look at the successes and failures of two people who can help you deal with the pressures in *your* day-to-day life. This is a 'must read' book!"

**Dennis Rainey**
Director, Family Ministry


"*Managing Stress in Marriage* is a breath of fresh air. For years I've wanted to hear Bill and Vonette share their insights on a marriage that has been a model for Dottie and me—and now we have the tremendous benefits of their lives together."

**Josh McDowell**
Josh McDowell Ministry

# MANAGING STRESS IN MARRIAGE

## Bill & Vonette Bright

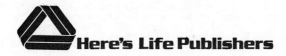

Here's Life Publishers

First Printing, April 1990


Published by
HERE'S LIFE PUBLISHERS, INC.
P. O. Box 1576
San Bernardino, CA 92402

**Library of Congress Cataloging-in-Publication Data**
Bright, Bill.
   Managing stress in marriage : help for couples on the fast track / Bill and
Vonette Bright.
   p.      cm.
   ISBN 0-89840-272-7
   1. Marriage—Religious aspects—Christianity. 2. Marriage—Psychological
aspects. 3. Stress (Psychology). I. Bright, Vonette Z. II. Title.
   BV835.B69   1990
   248.8'44—dc 20                          89-24585
                                              CIP


Scripture quotations designated NIV are from *The Holy Bible: New International Version,* ©
1973, 1978, 1984 by the International Bible Society. Used by permission of Zondervan Bible
Publishers. Scripture quotations designated TLB are from *The Living Bible,* © 1971 by Tyn-
dale House Publishers, Wheaton, Illinois. Scripture quotations designated NASB are from *The
New American Standard Bible,* © The Lockman Foundation 1960, 1962, 1963, 1968, 1971,
1972, 1975, 1977. Scripture quotations designated RSV are from *The Holy Bible: Revised Standard Version,* © 1952. Published by Thomas Nelson & Sons, New York. Scripture quotations
designated TEV are from *The Good News Bible: Today's English Version,* © 1966, 1971, 1976
by the American Bible Society. Published by Thomas Nelson Publishers, Nashville, Ten-
nessee.


**For More Information, Write:**
*L.I.F.E.*—P.O. Box A399, Sydney South 2000, Australia
*Campus Crusade for Christ of Canada*—Box 300, Vancouver, B.C., V6C 2X3, Canada
*Campus Crusade for Christ*—Pearl Assurance House, 4 Temple Row, Birmingham, B2 5HG, England
*Lay Institute for Evangelism*—P.O. Box 8786, Auckland 3, New Zealand
*Campus Crusade for Christ*—P.O. Box 240, Raffles City Post Office, Singapore 9117
*Great Commission Movement of Nigeria*—P.O. Box 500, Jos, Plateau State Nigeria, West Africa
*Campus Crusade for Christ International*—Arrowhead Springs, San Bernardino, CA 92414, U.S.A.

*To our beloved sons Zac and Brad and our daughter-in-love Terry. And to all of the many staff of Campus Crusade for Christ who through the years have served the Lord as our personal associates and have helped to maximize our daily schedules, enabling us to have a more active and fruitful ministry individually and together. You know us so well and you have helped to make us what we are. We trust you are pleased with the product you have helped produce. You are dearly loved and greatly appreciated.*

# *Contents*

Acknowledgments . . . . . . . . . . . . . . . . . . . 9

### Part 1: Recognizing the Reality of Stress

1. The Uninvited Guest . . . . . . . . . . . . . . . 13
2. The Many Faces of Stress . . . . . . . . . . . . 22

### Part 2: Steps to Managing Stress in Marriage

*Step 1: Enter Into a Partnership*

3. The Stress of Sharing a Dream . . . . . . . . . 33
4. The Stress of Role Confusion . . . . . . . . . . 46
5. The Stress of Personality Differences . . . . . . 57
6. The Stress of Being an Entrepreneur . . . . . . 68
7. The Stress of Divided Loyalties . . . . . . . . . 81

*Step 2: Establish God-Centered Priorities*

8. The Throne Check . . . . . . . . . . . . . . . . 91
9. Agree on Stewardship Principles . . . . . . . .106

*Step 3: Utilize Stress-Reducers*

10. The Power of Praise . . . . . . . . . . . . . . .119
11. Intimacy Through Communication . . . . . . .128
12. Sex: God's Gift for Stress Relief . . . . . . . . .139

*Step 4: Handle the Stress of Family*

13. The Stress of Children . . . . . . . . . . . . . .151
14. Managing Family Crises . . . . . . . . . . . . .161

*Step 5: Prepare for the Golden Years*

15. The Empty Nest . . . . . . . . . . . . . . . . .171
16. Growing in Retirement . . . . . . . . . . . . .180

# Part 3: A Personal Word

17. Building a Home in a Pull-Apart World:
    A Word to Women From Vonette . . . . . . . . .193
18. Radical Lover—Intimate Leader:
    A Word to Men From Bill . . . . . . . . . . . .208
19. The World Awaits . . . . . . . . . . . . . . . .219
Notes . . . . . . . . . . . . . . . . . . . . . . .222

# Acknowledgments

Well, world, here it is –

... more than forty years of joyful, adventuresome life together, expressed in words and story revealing the principles that have kept our marriage vibrant, exciting and alive. We have endeavored to be honest, frank and practical to be of help to couples who want to stay together for a full and rewarding lifetime. To be honest, we feel embarrassed to share some of the intimacies, but we have been told they are needed to show that we're "real people."

Vonette and I are deeply grateful to God for giving us the opportunity to be involved together in a worldwide ministry for our dear Lord. The Holy Spirit has provided the glue that kept us together. And God alone deserves the honor and glory for any and all of our accomplishments.

Many have contributed to our growing insights and helped enrich our relationship with each other, but we are especially aware of the contributions made by the staff of Campus Crusade for Christ, who are the most important people in the world to us apart from our family. They help make so much of what we do possible. Many of our most exciting moments as a couple have been with our beloved staff.

This book has been a team effort involving Les Stobbe, president of Here's Life Publishers, and writers and researchers Don Tanner, Joette Whims and Barbara Fagan, who have spent many hours helping us with the manuscript to articulate what God has taught us about the joy of biblical marriage, making commitments to God and each other, and living each day in His presence and for His glory.

Special thanks also to our associates Steve Douglass, executive vice president of Campus Crusade for Christ; Judy Douglass, former editor of *Worldwide Challenge*; Dennis Rainey, director of Family Ministry; Mary Graham and Steve Sellers, associate directors of U.S. Ministries; Robert R. Thompson, General Counsel for Campus Crusade; and Erma Griswold, affectionately known as "Mrs. G," my longtime associate, for reading the manuscript and providing most helpful comments.

Thank you, all who have labored with us to make this book a reality. To God be the glory!

# Part 1

# Recognizing the Reality of Stress

# 1

# *The*
# *Uninvited Guest*

"Ladies and gentlemen, please remain in your seats and keep your seat belts fastened. We should be out of the storm in a few moments . . . "

The calm voice over the intercom was hardly reassuring as our Pan Am 707 pierced the fury of a storm during our flight from New York to Washington, D.C. The sky flashed as lightning forked its tongue, seemingly just inches away from the plane. Swirling winds tore at the plane's metal skin, and the aircraft bounced and shuddered in the turbulence.

I gripped Vonette's hand and turned to look at her strained face, letting my eyes drink in every beloved curve.

"I don't know how much longer the plane can endure this storm without breaking into pieces," I worried.

She nodded gravely, and I recalled our arrival at the airport in New York City from Amsterdam.

The sky had been ominous, with clouds hanging low and ponderous like the underbellies of a huge herd of cat-

tle. Neither of us paid more than passing attention to the
menacing weather as we disembarked.

We passed through customs as quickly as possible,
then transferred to the domestic terminal to locate the gate
for our sixty-five-minute flight to Washington where we
both had meetings set for the next day. By the time our
plane was scheduled to depart, however, the heavy clouds
burst into a downpour. The weather quickly worsened into
an electrical storm that grounded our aircraft. Vonette and
I, together with our son Brad and Dr. David Hock Tey,
director of Chinese Ministries for Campus Crusade for
Christ, settled in the boarding area to wait for the weather
to clear.

After considerable delay, the rain stopped and the
loudspeaker announced our departure. We gathered our
carry-on baggage and hurried to the gate, anxious to be on
our way. Before we finished boarding, however, the rain
started again.

Vonette eased into a window seat, and I strapped
myself in beside her. David chose the aisle seat next to me
so we could go over some ministry matters during the flight.
Brad settled directly across the aisle from him.

The plane took off smoothly, knifing its way through
the light rain into the thick gauze of clouds. Forgetting the
weather, David and I immersed ourselves in conversation.
Hardly fifteen minutes into our flight, however, the aircraft
began to lift and drop like the rise and fall of a breath-taking
roller coaster ride. Nervous passengers tittered throughout
the cabin. Leaning over Vonette to peer out the window, I
saw lightning streak again and again across the sky. With
each threatening bolt, the sky seemed to explode in bril-
liant flashes. We seemed to be in the heart of a ball of white
fire.

The 707 began to twist—first to the right, then to the

left—in the increasing fury. The shaky laughter around me faded into an eerie silence, broken only by the calm voice of the flight attendant. Through the windows we could see the wings flapping almost like those of a giant bird struggling frantically against a violent downdraft.

Beside me, David began rocking and chanting in his Oriental fashion, "O God. O Lord, save us. O God. O Lord, save us."

Vonette leaned toward me, and I felt the gentle pressure of her hand entwined in mine. Softly, we began praying, our words flowing together in supplication to our precious Savior.

Convinced that our aircraft could not survive the turbulence much longer, I tenderly said goodbye to my dear Vonette and she to me. Then, together, we told our wonderful Lord that we were ready to meet Him if He desired.

Immediately, we sensed a peace flowing over us like a gentle river, a stillness that quieted our fears as though we had just nestled into a serene cocoon. Vonette's hand relaxed in mine, and we leaned over David to reassure Brad. He had heard us saying our goodbyes.

"We love you, son," I said solemnly. Vonette echoed my statement with a mother's compassionate gaze.

He smiled wanly, his face ashen.

The prayers and consolations of our little group were the only sounds coming from the cabin. Suddenly, I thought of how the Lord Jesus had calmed the winds and water on the sea when His disciples feared that their boat would capsize during another violent storm. Knowing His power and love for all His children, I prayed aloud, "Lord, You are the God of all creation. You control the laws of nature. You quieted the storm on the Sea of Galilee. Quiet this storm!"

Immediately the rain and the turbulence stopped.

Vonette stared at me in amazement, then smiled slightly. "Now, why didn't we pray that prayer earlier?"

I squeezed her hand and grinned back. Our fragile plane flew on, threading through the thick darkness abandoned by the lightning. You can be sure that Vonette and I continued to thank and praise the Lord for hearing our prayers and saving our lives. Hours later, the pilot skillfully brought the plane down in a smooth landing at a freight terminal in Norfolk, a long way from our destination. The flight that should have lasted sixty-five minutes had become a four-hour nightmare of blind flying and had taken us to a small airport in Virginia.

We learned later that the lightning had knocked a huge hole in the fuselage near the cockpit, destroying all the radar equipment. The pilot said this was the most violent storm he had ever experienced in millions of miles of flying.

Vonette and I made it to our meetings in Washington the next morning on time, but it required traveling by bus the rest of the night.

## High-Stress Lifestyle

We have experienced many stresses during our more than forty years of marriage, although not all have been as dramatic as this flight. As cofounders and leaders of the international movement of Campus Crusade for Christ, we live fast-paced and exciting lives. Yet, this lifestyle can put extraordinary strain on our relationship. Things like extensive travel, hectic schedules, living and rearing a family in a fish bowl environment, managing the tension between ministry and family, and the writing of many books and articles all increase the pressure.

Many couples experiencing similar lifestyles at times wonder how their relationship can survive.

Some marriages, I have observed, seem like the quiet waters of a lake at sunrise, not a ripple disturbing the surface. Others, particularly those of couples on the run, more closely resemble the Sea of Galilee, unpredictable and decidedly stormy at times.

The media and some Christians would like us to believe that all marriages should resemble the quiet lake. Thus when a couple's relationship takes on the characteristics of the stormy Sea of Galilee, many spouses decide that those periods are simply too tough to handle. They conclude that the external and internal stresses are more than they can bear, and opt out of their marriage.

We are writing this book to tell you that a high-stress marriage can succeed — and succeed gloriously; that even the stresses of leading an international ministry or any other stressful endeavor can be turned into marriage-strengtheners.

And there are stresses in every marriage, though Jesus does enable us to manage or overcome stress when we fully trust and obey Him.[1]

## The Uninvited Guest

In fact, you could call stress "the uninvited guest" because when you least expect him, he appears in your midst, at your table, and interrupts your most intimate moments.

Have you ever felt invaded when you opened the door to someone from out of town who was totally unexpected? Whether the uninvited guest was a relative, a friend, or the friend of a friend, he would force us into special efforts because of the same factors: We do not expect the visit; we are not mentally and emotionally prepared for the visit; it interrupts planned activity; and the visitor may create relationship problems in our home. All of these factors are intricately involved in a high-stress marriage as well, making stress management an essential ingredient in an intimate and loving relationship.

Let's take a brief look at how stress in marriage resembles that uninvited guest.

## 1. Stress Comes Unexpectedly

Probably the key factor affecting our response to stress is its unexpectedness. After all, we think, stress may be common in the marriage where one or both are not believers, but for Christians? If Christ is resident in us and we are filled with the Holy Spirit, why should we experience stress?

Yet even the most dedicated Christian spouses encounter this uninvited guest in their home.

A few years ago, I had the privilege of traveling all over the world helping to launch city-wide and country-wide campaigns to encourage millions of Christians to help saturate the world with the gospel through a strategy called Here's Life World. One of my stops was Sao Paulo, Brazil.

The first day, I met with our Brazilian staff to help formulate strategies for establishing Here's Life Brazil in all the major communities of the country. This and other conferences I would attend marked the beginning of a tour that would take me all over Latin America to help launch Here's Life Latin America. I was excited about the trip and the potential of working with these godly Christians to enable millions to hear the gospel in this part of the world.

Late that night, however, I received a call from Vonette who was at home in Arrowhead Springs. Her voice sounded apprehensive.

"Honey, I haven't been feeling well . . . "

"What's wrong?"

"I went to the doctor, and he took some tests. Bill . . .

I have a large tumor," she choked. "He wants to operate right away!"

"I'll take the next flight home!" I exclaimed.

"No, Bill, you'd better continue with your meetings. I know how crucial the Here's Life campaign is."

"But I want to be with you," I insisted.

As we discussed the situation over the telephone, I felt torn between my love and deep concern for Vonette and my burden for millions of people whom we longed to reach for Christ. But I could not be in two parts of the world at the same time. Which place should I choose? What would the Lord want me to do?

Once again, the uninvited guest had shown up at my door.

Stress is an unexpected element in all of our lives. No matter how much we try to prepare for it, stress usually catches us off guard. For couples on the fast track, however, the frequency and intensity of unexpected pressure can strain a relationship to the breaking point. How they react to high-pressure situations will make a lasting impact on their marriage. In a later chapter, we will tell you how we experienced God's grace to cope when Vonette faced surgery.

## 2. Stress Interrupts Planned Activities

When stress comes into our lives as the uninvited guest, he usually intrudes on our daily routine and makes unreasonable demands on our time and energy.

Bill and I had an experience of this nature last weekend. Our children were home visiting on a Saturday when Bill suggested that we entertain guests for dinner Sunday afternoon. Thinking of the preparations I would have to make and of my already full schedule, I objected immediately.

"Well, now wait! I'm not sure I want to work that hard, and I had planned on spending a quiet evening with the family."

"As I said, I don't think it's a good idea to have guests on Sunday," Bill grinned in quick retreat.

He has this disarming way about him.

Then I realized our family would enjoy visiting with these wonderful people. So I considered how much time I had to devote to fixing the meal and decided to start the preparations right away. By pacing myself, I could get it all done without destroying any of my plans. We did have guests, and enjoyed a lovely visit.

And Vonette prepared such a delicious dinner that I went off my diet for that one meal!

Interruptions can cause friction in a high-stress marriage, especially when they come one right after another. When each of us is carrying a heavy schedule and is involved in many activities, intrusions may cause our entire day to run behind or make it impossible to do everything we planned. Then stress can build until it causes conflict, illness or depression. How we handle interruptions immensely affects our marriage relationship.

### 3. Stress Can Create Relationship Problems

When pressures build, the natural reaction of spouses is to take the frustration out on each other. A critical spirit, outbursts of anger, hurt feelings, and many other destructive emotions follow to damage the intimacy between a husband and wife.

When Liz's babysitter quit with only two days' notice, Liz brought the dilemma to her husband Ralph. But he didn't respond the way she wanted. Instead, he drew back behind his newspaper and abandoned Liz to find her own day care solution.

"I was angry," Liz explained. "The children's welfare was *our* problem, not just mine! I still had dinner to cook and three loads of laundry to do that evening. I couldn't face yet another burden on my time and energy. So I lashed out at Ralph."

## Looking Ahead

When "the uninvited guest" appears at your table, how do you handle his intrusion? Does his presence change the way you relate to your spouse? Will his frequent arrivals turn your relationship into a shambles? Is there a godly way to manage his effect on your marriage?

By now you probably are ready to tell your own story of unexpected stress. In fact, you may be experiencing a truly stressful situation right now. We are here to tell you that there is hope.

In the coming pages, we want to share with you the secrets we have learned that will help you come out on the other side of the stress with a stronger relationship with the Lord and with your mate. You can learn as we have that the Lord is faithful even during the most stressful situation imaginable.

And do we have a few of those in case you'd like to compare notes!

Vonette and I discovered that when you put a "visionary" together with a "let's get things done" person in a marriage, that's a recipe for stress on a grand scale . . .

# 2

# *The Many Faces of Stress*

I received an urgent call from our international vice president, Bailey Marks, one morning this summer before Vonette and I left on a trip to the Philippines to meet with all of our continental leaders.

"Bill, security forces in Manila suspect a Communist threat against Campus Crusade during our up-coming DOA[1] meetings in Baguio City and the Lausanne conference in Manila. I called you because, as president, you would be a special target."

"What's the situation there?" I asked.

"Communist terrorists are accelerating their campaign to overthrow the government. Because of our evangelistic commitment to proclaim the gospel, Campus Crusade could be one of their major targets."

"What do the security forces want me to do?"

"Well, Bill, they strongly recommend a police escort to and from the conferences. And they want to station armed guards outside your hotel room at all times. Should

I give them the go-ahead?"

I leaned forward in my chair. "I'll discuss this with Vonette and call you back later."

I weighed the seriousness of the threat and prayed for wisdom. Traveling the world, Vonette and I frequently face danger because of our high visibility. Yet we cannot function at our maximum in our positions of leadership and live in fear. We feel we must go wherever our Lord leads us—even if it might involve danger.

Contemplating the threats in Manila, I sighed deeply. More bothersome precautions. And pressure. The possibility of unknown assailants and the presence of our guards would cause uneasiness for everyone around us.

Later that night, I discussed Bailey's call with Vonette.

I didn't understand the seriousness of the situation until Bill mentioned Communist terrorists. We realized that if someone planned to attack, there was not much the security forces could do. Yet we didn't want to take unnecessary risks.

Following our meeting with the directors of affairs in Baguio, we would have to travel four hours by bus through what was believed to be terrorist territory to Manila for the Lausanne II Congress on Evangelism. We considered the security problem, and I suggested that Bill return to the United States immediately after our meetings. He agreed.

Later, when I returned Bailey's call, I explained what Vonette and I had decided. "So we would prefer the least amount of security possible," I concluded.

"You realize the danger?"

"Yes," I replied.

Bailey sighed. "Okay. I'll make the arrangements here."

Our trip to the Philippines went without incident. When I left Vonette to fly home, I took comfort in the knowledge that our Lord would protect her. Even so, I wished she were with me.

Vonette and I, as well as you and your spouse, cannot escape the effects of stress. When stress is our constant companion, how can we live simply from day to day and relax and rely on our Lord's love and care? How does depending on God for every facet of our lives help us handle the myriad pressures of our busy lifestyles?

## Understanding Stress

To handle the pressures in our lives successfully, we need to clearly understand the meaning and function of stress.

Dr. Gary Collins, a Christian psychologist and authority on stress, calls stress the wear and tear of living which each of us experiences as the result of the pressures of life.

Stress in itself is neither good nor bad; it's what we make of it that really counts. "When it motivates us to action," Dr. Collins says, "stress can be good." That's why our heart pounds and our blood pressure rises when we receive a promotion. Or why we felt out of breath when our sweetheart agreed to be our wife. "But," Dr. Collins warns, "when stress puts our bodies under prolonged physical and emotional pressure, then the very things that might have been stimulating and fun become destructive and unpleasant instead."[2]

The writer of Proverbs seems to affirm this: "Anxious hearts are very heavy."[3] Or as another translation of this verse says, "Heaviness in the heart of man *maketh it stoop.*"[4]

Often we fail to see the difference between stress and its cause. According to authors Bill and Deana Blackburn, stress is "the pressure we feel from positive or negative events in our lives (called stressors) and the effect these events have on us."[5] My stress is the reaction I *feel* toward the "stressor" or source of my feeling.

Let me illustrate: Many of the hotel rooms at Arrowhead Springs have balconies from which guests can view the panorama of San Bernardino below. How relaxing it feels to stand near the balustrade on one of those verandas, three or four stories up, and gaze at the beautiful postcard scene.

I would feel differently standing there without that railing, however. My attention would be drawn toward the ground and how easily I could fall.

The stressor in this example is the distance I could fall. The stress is my fear of falling—my response to the danger. Whatever the pressure source, a clear understanding of this difference will help us to handle our responses positively.

## Faces of Stress

All marriages, particularly those of ministry leaders, professionals and business executives, experience a varied pattern of stress which, if not attended to, can wreck a marriage and invalidate one's ministry.

We know well how a busy lifestyle adds extraordinary pressure to a relationship. The stress and strain comes in innumerable forms and at unpredictable times. We have discovered that "the uninvited guest" of stress truly has many faces.

Imagine that the uninvited guest suddenly appears at your doorstep. He pushes past you and makes himself comfortable without waiting for you to ask him in. Realizing that he plans to stay for weeks, maybe even months, you study his habits and get to know him well so you can adapt your schedule to his demands.

To predict his every move, you memorize every line of his face and take note of all his expressions. Then one morning, he walks pompously to the breakfast table with a different face. Dismayed, you realize that your guest has been wearing a mask. So you begin to study his new face. But before you figure him out, he changes again.

No matter how quickly you get to know his new faces, he switches. His ever-changing presence keeps your entire family off-balance trying to adjust.

This is how stress affects couples on the fast track. The uninvited guest appears in so many forms and in such varied patterns that he drains them of their energy and coping abilities. This leads to stress exhaustion and even more pressure.

The many faces worn by the uninvited guest personify the pressures of a dual career, a fast-paced schedule, being on call, and living in a fish bowl environment. We have seen these faces many times; the uninvited guest is a persistent visitor.

## Excess Stress

Stress as an essential survival mechanism is healthy. But when we experience too much of it, the excess stress is potentially dangerous to our health and our relationships. Some people, however, thrive on the excess stress. Like drug addicts needing a fix, they keep themselves under constant pressure to help them accomplish their tasks. But stress has a cumulative effect.[6] When one difficult situation after another buffets us, tension builds faster than our responses can handle, and breakdown can occur.

Is excess stress an unavoidable part of our lives? Do we have to let the uninvited guest disturb the tranquility of our homes? Definitely not. We choose the amount of stress we feel by deciding the way we will respond to the causes of stress in our lives.

In spite of the divorce statistics and stressors that work against us, I remain optimistic about marriage. I believe we can develop response patterns that will deepen the intimacy in our relationships.

Years ago, my dearly beloved pastor, Dr. Louis Evans, Sr., used to say: "Marriage is God's idea and only with His help can we work it out with joy." In the coming chapters we will share positive steps you can take to prevent "the uninvited guest" from turning your life into turmoil. And we will show you how to manage his intrusion under the power of the Holy Spirit.

## Steps to Recognizing and Managing Stress

As leaders of a worldwide ministry, Vonette and I have observed and experienced the varied patterns of stress that many ministry leaders, professionals and business executives share. We have learned how stress can unite and strengthen the relationship of a busy couple.

In the following chapters, we will show you how the uninvited guest shaped our lifetime of ministry together. We will suggest five steps for recognizing and managing stress that will enable you to strengthen your marriage and achieve greater intimacy.

Our Lord has not promised us a stress-free life. Some of the heroes of the Bible lived under harsh circumstances. David watched two of his sons rebel against his leadership; Joseph was unjustly accused of attacking Potiphar's wife; the apostle Paul endured beatings and imprisonment. Yet in all their difficulties, faithful men and women triumphed through the power of God.

    As Christians, we have an eternal advantage over the world. We can change the way we respond to both good and bad situations through the power of the Holy Spirit. When our lives are based on the wisdom of His Word and a day-by-day walk with Him, we can learn to be victorious through all of our stresses and still live a full and joyful life with our mate.

# Part 2

# Steps to Managing Stress in Marriage

# *Step 1*

## Enter Into a Partnership

*God established marriage as a partnership.
But couples must consciously commit themselves
to the Lord and to each other, and remain alert
to any threat to their union.*

# 3

# *The Stress of Sharing a Dream*

I glanced at my watch once again. 1:25 P.M. Five minutes later than the last time I checked. Where could Bill have gone?

I was sitting alone in a hot car in the empty parking lot of Hollywood Presbyterian Church. I had not seen Bill since that older couple had pulled him aside after Sunday school to talk privately. Church had been over for more than an hour. And as a young bride, I felt awkward about barging in on their huddled group—wherever they were.

The afternoon sun was beating on the windshield. But the flush of anger creeping up my cheeks made me even hotter than the stuffy car. I tried to put the puzzle together.

I had waited patiently so that Bill and I could walk to the church service together. Finally, I had gone to the service alone. All during the sermon, I had craned my neck searching for him. But he hadn't come. After the service, he was still nowhere to be found. As the crowd thinned and cars were pulling out of the parking lot onto Hollywood Boulevard, I decided to wait in our car rather than stand on the steps of the locked church—alone. I could have walked to our home only ten blocks away, but the thought of walking uphill on a hot day didn't appeal to me.

So here I sat. Irritated. Feeling totally forsaken. *Why is he spending so much time with this couple? What's so private about their conversation that they couldn't include me? At least Bill could have excused himself and told me where he was going!* I checked the time once more. Two o'clock. *Maybe he left with that couple and forgot I was here. Certainly not very considerate! What does he think I'm doing, anyway?*

Suddenly, the car door opened. There stood Bill with a sheepish grin on his face. "Been waiting long?" he asked lamely as he slid behind the wheel.

I turned my face away from his.

"You're crying, Vonette," he empathized softly.

My throat tightened.

"I'm sorry, honey. Time got away from me." He leaned over and put his arm around me.

"Where have you been? How could you *possibly* keep me waiting like this?" I choked. "I had no idea what happened to you."

He tried to wipe away my tears. "I'm so sorry. We just got involved talking. It was one of those things I didn't have control over. Both of those people can really talk! They needed my counsel about a very serious matter."

"It just better not happen again, Bill Bright! I might not be waiting next time," I said flatly. "Let's go home."

We drove the short distance from the church to our home in the Hollywood hills in silence. Closing the front door behind us, he took me in his arms. "Honey, I love you. This was all a mistake. It won't happen again."

He helped me prepare our meal, but I couldn't shake

myself of the hurt and resentment, nor hide my feelings.

"Why are you still angry?" he asked over lunch.

I hesitated before answering. "It's not just that you ignored me this morning. I'm not happy with the way things are going in our marriage. Most of the time you're so considerate and thoughtful. And I appreciate the way you include me in some of your business decisions. But other times, you're very insensitive. You don't consider my feelings when you get busy with other people. And when you plan your schedule, you assume I'll just fit in somewhere."

Bill frowned. "Do you think we're doing too much? Should I cut back?"

I shook my head. "It's not exactly that. I feel left out. Just an add-on to your life."

He took my hand. "Why don't we sit down after lunch and decide what is important to both of us? We could make a list of what we really want out of life."

I nodded my head slowly, not sure what good that would do.

Suddenly Bill sat straight up in his chair. "I know what we could do! Let's make a contract. Just between you and me and the Lord. So it's not your way or my way but *our* way—serving the Lord together."

As a businessman, Bill had signed hundreds of contracts. From his perspective, it seemed reasonable to make an agreement between us and the Lord, too. I felt myself catching his fervor. "You mean, sign it and everything?"

He started to clear the table. "Yes. Let's do it this afternoon. Let's write down exactly what we want out of life. Our lifetime goals. And put the contract where we both can see it to remind us that we are committed to working together."

"Yes, let's do it," I agreed with all my heart.

Later that afternoon, we did write and sign a contract, surrendering our lives completely and irrevocably to the Lord and to each other. That stressful situation helped us realize how much we needed the Lord and that apart from Him our marriage could not survive. By surrendering everything to the Lord, we created in our marriage a partnership that we have enjoyed more and more each year. That contract has been the foundation for our lives and ministry since the spring of 1951.

## Marriage Is a Partnership

Though God ultimately holds the husband accountable for the leadership in the home, Vonette and I strongly believe that marriage is a partnership between equal participants.[1] We believe the scriptural truth that we are to become one,[2] and we try to model this in our relationship.

To establish partnership in marriage, *couples must consciously commit themselves to the Lord and to each other, and stay alert to any threat to their union.*

I really believe this commitment begins with the attitude of the husband. When he truly understands the importance of loving his wife as Christ loved the church,[3] he will not demand to be served by his wife. Instead, he will ask himself, "How can I help her be God's maximum person? How can I help her enjoy life more and live less stressfully?"

Many of the counseling problems I encounter started when the man insisted on his rights. And that attitude often prevails in Christian homes.

God intended marriage to be the closest human bond. All too often, however, the stressors that invade a marriage pull spouses apart. Let me suggest three steps you can take to protect your partnership from these pressures.

## 1. Surrender Your Marriage to God

To grow together, you and your spouse must yield yourselves to the Lord. This includes time to pray and discuss the Scriptures together. With this spiritual foundation, your lives will begin to blend. You will learn to cope with the difficulties in your relationship—the irritations, frustrations and differences between you. As you walk together in spiritual partnership, you will surmount the crises and hectic pace of your lives and grow in intimacy.

Tragically, many spouses do not share such spiritual commitment. Neglecting prayer and the study of God's Word, they depend on church attendance or casual Christian fellowship for their spiritual health. Eventually, their lack of commitment to the Lord filters into their marriage.

Perhaps you are experiencing this in your relationship. What do you do? I encourage you to pray for your partner. Find a convenient time to discuss his/her spiritual commitment. Don't be judgmental. Graciously, lovingly encourage your mate to take an active role in your spiritual partnership.

God understands you and your mate perfectly and can empower you with His Holy Spirit to build your spiritual relationship. Later in this book, we will share practical guidelines on how you can live the Spirit-filled life day-by-day.

## 2. Agree to Walk Together

When a couple agree to walk together, they accept each other's beliefs, hopes and desires, and they work through the expectations each brings to the relationship. This is a life-time process. Vonette and I are still discovering ways to improve our walk.

Because we believe in this concept so much, we insist that our Campus Crusade staff couples serve equally. Unless they have children, both partners are expected to be on the job. Neither spouse can work at another full- or part-time job, unless he is a volunteer. We also encourage couples at our International School of Theology to take marital training along with their theological studies. This has vitalized the ministries of our graduating students.

## 3. Share a Dream

Sharing each other's dreams is vital to partnership. Vonette and I have had many dreams through the years, but as an expression of our love for the Lord, our deep gratitude for all that He has done for us and our desire to obey Him, the single most important objective of our lives is to help fulfill the Great Commission of our Lord—the vision God gave me not long after we signed our contract.

Along with others, I had been sharing my faith on the UCLA and USC campuses for some time as a representative of our church, but with little success. One day Dr. Henrietta Mears, the Christian education director at Hollywood Presbyterian Church, presented a challenge that revitalized my ministry. She had just returned from a world tour and had seen the devastation left by World War II in Europe.

"The world is on fire!" she exclaimed. "Evil is rampant and people are hurting. Jesus Christ is what the world needs. I'm convinced that we need to make an impact on the whole world, not just here . . . "

As she shared her vision for the world, I began to catch her enthusiasm. But how and where would we start?

I thought of all the young, fresh faces I met on campus. Then it dawned on me: They could be the greatest resource for changing the world. They were the leadership of tomorrow. They *were* tomorrow.

At the time, I was operating my own fancy foods business and attending Fuller Theological Seminary. That evening, I stayed up until midnight preparing for a Greek exam with Hugh Brom, a fellow student.

Suddenly God began speaking to me—not audibly, but just as real. My heart burst with a sense of the Lord's presence.

It was as if a huge canvas of the world were spread before me. Like an artist's hand sketching a sky, mountains, streams and brooks, the painting only showed the high points, not the details. I sensed that the Lord was showing me a broad plan for taking the gospel to the whole world. I was to invest my life in helping to fulfill the Great Commission in this generation. I was to begin by helping to win and disciple the students of the world for Christ. How to do this was not spelled out in detail. Today, nearly forty years later, the Master Artist is still filling in the details on that canvas. The worldwide student ministry has spawned scores of other ministries designed to help fulfill the Great Commission.

Bill awakened me early in the morning, hardly able to contain himself. He was bubbling over with enthusiasm and joy. Groggily, I sat up in bed and mumbled, "Let me get up, and I'll prepare your breakfast."

"Honey, I don't need any breakfast." His intense enthusiasm overcame my desire to sink back into the pillows. Bill bustled out of the room. Springing out of bed, I slipped my robe from a hanger.

I found him standing in the kitchen, tears rolling down his cheeks.

He spoke slowly without looking at me. His voice quivered.

"Last night while I was studying, God spoke to me. Never have I felt His presence like that before! It happened so quickly. God has called me . . . God has called *us* to help take the gospel to the entire world. And He wants us to start by reaching students on the college campus."

Pulling out a chair, he sat down. Before him were his open text books. Closing the top one, he declared, "I'm dropping out of school. What God has told me to do is far more important than my final month of seminary."

Everything he shared to this point was beautiful; now he seemed to be over-reacting. Imagine throwing away five years of study at Princeton and Fuller seminaries with all the credentials that would soon be in his hands!

"Honey, you only have a few more units left," I gasped.

"But I can relate to students and laymen better as a lay person and business leader than as an ordained pastor," he insisted. "We're going to live by faith, Vonette. I want to sell the businesses and trade in that convertible for something modest. We're going to have to move closer to the campus."

Suddenly, I envisioned a gauge where the needle had moved from the normal zone into the red. But having watched my mother interact with my Dad, I knew better than to say anything while he was so impassioned.

Walking back into the bedroom, I felt the weight of such a radical change. *He's out in the kitchen doing a backstroke in ecstasy while I'm under water unable to breathe.*

Bill's dream seemed too big for me. His decision would mean a complete change of lifestyle for us. My mind raced. *I'm not the right wife for Bill. I could never accept the sacrifice. There are other women far more mature.*

I was not ready to give up the financial security which Bill had provided. I wanted to buy nice things and live the good life. I wanted a baby with bottles of milk in the refrigerator, not just a cold formula of faith.

One afternoon, after several days of trying to convince Bill of other alternatives of combining business and ministry, I sank to my knees and buried my face in the white chenille bedspread. "Oh, Lord," I cried, "if Bill is right, and this is right, I pray that You will give me a heart to respond."

Though my heart was filled with praise and thanksgiving to the Lord for this remarkable revelation, I still needed the counsel of more mature Christians. The next day I went to see one of my favorite seminary professors, Dr. Wilbur Smith, world famous Bible teacher, scholar and author of many books. As I shared with him what God had revealed to me, he got out of his chair and paced back and forth in his office, saying again and again, "This is of God. This is of God. I want to help you. Let me think and pray about it."

The next morning when I arrived for his eight o'clock class in English Bible, Dr. Smith called me out of the classroom into a little counseling room and handed me a piece of paper. On it he had scribbled the letters "CCC," after which he had written "Campus Crusade for Christ." He explained that God had provided the name for my vision.

I wasn't enthusiastic. Over the next few days, I exaggerated the matter of "living by faith." What if Bill bought an enormous striped tent to hold his crowd? I envisioned that he would put it in a lot by the campus with a "CCC" flag suspended from the center pole. And I would have to pass out gospel tracts at the entrance flap. Sometimes I imagined us in a single basement room reading Scriptures by kerosene lamp.

I wanted to share Bill's dream. But the changes and sacrifices his new life demanded would bring far more pressure than I thought I could handle.

I had a college degree and was teaching a course of

study I had written in the Los Angeles city schools. Eleanor Kalamus, who wrote the weekly newspaper column, "Glorify Yourself," was extracting chapters from this course for her column in the Hearst newspaper chain. Mrs. Kalamus was eager for my manuscript to be published, since in response to the column they already had eight thousand orders for a yet-to-be developed book.

Would I have to abandon everything I wanted to do to follow Bill? Should I accept his vision and become his partner?

Sharing each other's dreams leads to the purest form of partnership. The intimacy and love produced by sharing a dream pays tremendous dividends. It took some time for me to realize and accept this. Now, I was standing on the brink of a decision that would change the rest of our lives.

Bill filled his days with plans for the new ministry. His next move was to look for an advisory board of outstanding men and women of God to counsel him in the establishment of this ministry.

Bill also invited people to pray around the clock that God would do a unique work on the UCLA campus. He began to recruit and train interested students as teams to join us in visiting various fraternities and sororities, dormitories, and other groups on the campus. The teams, of which I was a part, presented personal testimonies of their faith in Christ. After their testimonies, Bill gave a brief message explaining who Christ is, why He came and how to know Him personally.

Meanwhile, I was occupied with my own work as a teacher. I took pleasure in seeing my ideas implemented into programs that influenced my students. Each day I would come home from work and share what was going on in my classroom. Bill was just as exuberant about what was happening on the UCLA campus. At that point our differing dreams could have really divided us.

Personally, I was of two minds. I wanted Bill to acknowledge my career potential. But at the same time I didn't want him to develop his ministry without me.

As he would describe his strategy for evangelism, I sensed an invisible altar waiting somewhere ahead. Gradually, the Lord Jesus answered my prayer for a "heart to respond," and I became willing to put my sacrifices on that altar — my master's degree, my career, my book manuscript.

Bill's loving assurances and warmth made my struggle easier. I would never be happy, I realized, outside his dream. And in all these years, I haven't regretted my decision to merge my dreams with his.

Not only has my life been richer, but just like Abraham when he offered up Isaac, the Lord has multiplied everything I gave up many times over. And He has enabled me to see and experience more than I ever could have done alone.

Sharing our dreams has given Vonette and me a sense of oneness. In working together, we have developed a purpose to our relationship. We have discovered refuge and release in our closeness. We have challenged each other to grow through our failures and successes.

Most couples do not have opportunity to work together as we do. But all can choose a dream worthy of their united effort. Ask the Holy Spirit to help you catch the vision of partnership and experience oneness. Let your dream draw you and your spouse together. As you share each other's dreams, you will experience the joy and satisfaction of achieving something of eternal value.

## The Stress of Sharing a Dream

Sharing a dream brings its own stress, however. Seldom do a husband and wife begin their life together with the same dream for their marriage and for themselves. The stress is accentuated when both are committed to all-out service for Jesus Christ, either vocationally or avocationally.

A couple's interests can be so different that they must work hard at appreciating and contributing to each other's objectives. Or their dreams may be so alike that they find themselves competing. At certain times in a relationship, one partner may believe that his dream is more crucial than his spouse's. Misguided priorities also create conflict. I'm sure you can think of many other stresses in sharing a dream.

Bill is not only a dreamer but a mover and a shaker. When he has a dream, he puts his entire body, soul and spirit into it. That sometimes causes tension for me.

One of the hardest things for me to face, for example, is our schedules. Although Bill and I usually travel together, we sometimes find ourselves on opposite sides of the world. Others must manage our calendars for us. In an organization as large as Campus Crusade, scheduling oversights sometimes complicate and compromise our time together.

Yesterday, for example. While we were working on this manuscript, Bill's assistant put his calendar on our working table. As I scanned it, I was shocked.

"Bill! Do you realize that we don't have *one* free weekend for nearly five months?"

He grinned sheepishly, "How did you let that happen?"

Ignoring his humor, I said firmly, "This schedule has gotten out of hand."

Immediately, we set about building time in the schedule for ourselves.

Stress can build between a husband and wife if he or she does not consider the other when taking on a new project. If either Bill or I decide to accept a major responsibility, we usually talk the situation over before making a final decision. How will this new responsibility affect us? Will it cause a conflict in our schedules? Does it really help us fulfill our shared objectives? Will this opportunity help us to fulfill the Great Commission? I try to evaluate my daily activities in light of this goal. This is what partnership in sharing a dream is all about.

As you begin your partnership, discover your dreams and build your marriage on them. Make sure these visions are worthy of the calling the Lord has given you. Whether your dreams are simple and down-to-earth or grandiose and complicated, embrace your mate's aspirations with a sense of encouragement and excitement. Dedicate yourself to serving the Lord and your partner for life. Then you will experience marriage in its fullest sense.

## For Reflection, Discussion and Action

1. Amos 3:3 asks, "Can two walk together, unless they are agreed?" How can you and your spouse improve your walk together? Discuss with your partner.

2. How can you and your spouse better fit in with each other's ideals, goals and plans?

3. What dream do you and your spouse share? How have you verbally expressed that dream to your mate?

# 4

# *The Stress of Role Confusion*

I had high expectations for our life together when I married Vonette. I wanted to build her a castle in prestigious Bel Air where I would be the king and she the queen. We would live the good life, raise lovely children and travel the world together. With the success I was having in my business, I looked forward to providing for her a truly prosperous lifestyle.

Although I intended to keep her abreast of my business dealings in a general way, I never expected her to be central to my success. Nor to achieve on her own. I pictured her simply as my wife, the mother of our children, and the keeper of our beautiful "castle."

I brought similar expectations to our marriage. Marrying a prosperous businessman, I assumed Bill would provide for me at least on the level to which I was accustomed.

I didn't want an active part in Bill's business affairs. Just before the wedding, he had asked my opinion about a

*46*

building he was selling. His request caught me off-guard. So I asked my uncle's advice. "Do you think Bill is making a good decision?"

"This man has made his business what it is without you," he counseled. "And I think he will continue to be successful without you. If I were you, I would not get involved in those kinds of questions."

I knew that my uncle provided well for my aunt. She knew little, however, about his business affairs. She just enjoyed the benefit of his success.

Most of the women I knew had a similar marital relationship. So I assumed that the role of a wife was to be passive and uninvolved in her husband's career. It surprised me that Bill expected more.

We didn't understand marital partnership in those days. For the first couple of years, I couldn't even sign our checks. I hadn't taken the time to put my name on our bank account. Even after I began teaching, I turned my paycheck over to Bill and expected him to handle our finances.

## Role Confusion

All couples enter marriage with expectations. These preconceptions can lead to confusion in the role a person should have in marriage. A role is a set of well-defined and expected behaviors. Couples bring all kinds of expectations to marriage, which set patterns in their relationship. Husbands and wives tend to relate to each other based on the way they saw their parents interact, or how they perceive their new roles.

As time goes on, circumstances in their lives change. The arrival of children, a job transfer, a new community, a new church—these create new expectations.

Modern society is much more complicated than that

of our parents. The changes that have taken place in American lifestyles since the 1950s have produced two major patterns for roles in families. "In the traditional breadwinner/housewife pattern," Joyce Portner explains, "the husband performs all of the employment functions and the wife virtually all of the household work functions. In the dual-employment pattern, husband and wife are each responsible for employment and household responsibilities."[1]

Consequently, roles today are harder to categorize. Where many spouses once understood exactly what the other would do in a situation, now they are unsure.

When you add the extra duties that a busy couple must balance, the chance for friction multiplies. Hectic lifestyles may upset normal expectations. You and your spouse may find yourselves functioning in areas where roles are not clearly defined. The resulting conflicts can threaten your oneness.

## The Stress of Role Confusion

Busy couples often find demands swirling and tugging at their relationship until they become exhausted and confused. "Why do you expect so much of me?" "How can I possibly do everything everyone wants?" "I feel terrible because I can't finish all the chores staring me in the face!"

Their self-image takes a beating and tempers flare when they can't balance responsibilities as they would like. Their once-peaceful home turns into a shouting arena. Their expectations begin to divide and separate them. They feel confused and unable to handle new situations and changing roles.

In our diversified world, the whirling transitions affecting us will keep us even more off-balance.

William Coleman writes, "Few areas in society are

moving as fast as the change in female roles. The steady and sure rise of women into management and leadership positions has introduced new dynamics into marriage relationships as well."[2] These changes and the resulting dual incomes frequently strain a relationship.

Is the plight of the busy couple hopeless? With our Lord's help and the couple's commitment to partnership, the stressors of role confusion can be turned into marriage strengtheners.

At one time, my changing role in the ministry put serious strain on our relationship.

The move to Arrowhead Springs in 1963 placed unusual demands on Bill. A man on our staff who didn't believe women should have a voice in business matters influenced him in decisions where my counsel was no longer sought.

I should have talked it out with Bill when I began to feel hurt, but I didn't. He made decision after decision without me, and I felt left out. Often I heard about changes long after they had been put into effect.

The situation finally came to a head when Bill and his administrator decided to place a print shop in the storage area of the hotel kitchen. They had taken over my area without a word to me. To do what they planned, they would have to cut into the kitchen vault where we kept our china, silver, and other important items.

At the time, I directed the kitchen and dining operation, oversaw the purchase of food, and planned the meals for our many conferences. Even though we didn't use all the kitchen and storage space, eventually we would need it. And I didn't want to end up working in cramped quarters.

One Sunday morning, while we were dressing for church, Bill casually mentioned their decision.

I objected. Emphatically.

"Well, the decision has been made and it is too late to change our plans now," he asserted.

I saw the determination in his eyes and heard it in his voice. Suddenly, all the resentment that had been building inside me erupted. "Okay, Bill Bright! I'll just leave! I'm not going to live where I have nothing to say about what goes on."

Neither of us said anything more. I grabbed a few items of clothing for the children and myself and marched the boys to the car.

"Okay," Bill said to my disappearing back, "If you feel so strongly, go on!"

I whisked the children into the car and slumped into the driver's seat. But I had no idea where to go. Tears welled in my eyes. What would I do?

Zac, our nine-year-old, quickly cut to the core. "Mother, this shows me just what kind of person you really are."

His words stung, and I shook my head. *This is so stupid, leaving like this.* But Bill hadn't begged me to come back, and my pride wouldn't let me back down. I didn't want to leave Bill, but I didn't want to continue in a relationship where there was no regard for my opinion. My mind raced quickly, trying to decide where to go.

Suddenly, Bill burst through the front door and strode to the front of the car. I would have had to run over him to drive away. "Don't go, Vonette," he pleaded loudly. He looked pathetic, and I felt ashamed.

I don't remember any other words but those. I had acted foolishly, but wasn't ready to admit it and give in. "I won't be treated like a woman who has no contribution to make," I fumed.

Bill apologized, then I did too. I stayed because he took the first step toward reconciling our problems. It took a real man of God to admit he was wrong, and this gave me the courage to confess my poor attitude.

Bill promised he would find another place to put the print shop. But as it turned out, we had no other option. I realized then that the real issue wasn't the print shop. It was my expectation. I had counted on Bill to include me in his decision-making. Unconsciously, he had diminished my part in the ministry.

This crisis showed us how vital partnership was to our marriage. That sad experience helped us be more aware of how we must work at walking together.

## How to Reduce Role-related Stress

In the early days of our marriage as we moved out of the business world into full-time ministry, Vonette became my colleague and co-laborer. In essence, my queen stepped down from her pedestal and took an active part in my life.

I remember our first sorority meeting at UCLA. It was at the Kappa Alpha Theta sorority, which was known as the "house of beautiful women." When I finished my message and presented the challenge to receive Christ, many girls remained behind to talk to us and ask questions. I was amazed to see such a large group of young women standing in line to express their desire to become Christians.

We invited the girls to join us the next evening for a meeting in our home nearby, and several of them brought their boyfriends. It was a memorable and exciting night. Many of the young men made decisions for Christ, too.

During a period of a few months, Vonette led about fifty women to the Lord. This opened my eyes to the impact she could have in my ministry. My expectations of Vonette changed rapidly.

My hopes for Bill changed drastically, too. I learned to be less dependent on him for my needs. As he took on more ministry and administrative responsibilities, he spent less time at home. I filled in the gaps and lessened my demands on him. And I learned to lean on the Lord more for my emotional needs and to let Bill do the same.

This in turn freed Bill to be more effective in his ministry. As each of us held fewer unrealistic expectations of the other, we gained confidence in our relationship.

Understanding the biblical order within the family is the key to reducing role-related stress.

Although God created husband and wife with equal worth and value, He designed for each a specific functional model. We believe the biblical pattern for the home is this: Husbands must love their wives as Christ loved the church, and wives should submit themselves to their husbands' leadership. The couple, in turn, should lovingly pass on their biblical values and their decisions to their children, who then are expected to obey their parents.[3]

We will share more on this biblical pattern in chapters 17 and 18.

Agreeing on how your God-given roles work in your marriage is essential. Through communication, you can come to terms with your roles and build understanding. You can discover each other's most vital needs and find ways to adapt to your unique situation.

A continuing process of evaluation will help you adjust to the changes in your marriage. Set aside specific times to reassess the roles in your relationship. How are they functioning? Discuss immediately any dissatisfaction you or your mate feels about any change.

Here are some guidelines to help you evaluate your roles to minimize stress.

## 1. Keep Your Roles Flexible

Sometimes a partner must fill many roles and function differently in each. Many women find it difficult, for example, to switch mindset from job to home. A leader by day, she may spend her time setting priorities and supervising employees. At home, however, she lets her husband assume the lead. A willingness to adjust to a different role makes the transition easier.

When I consider Bill's headship in whatever I do—even at work—it helps me keep my home and ministry in perspective. Not that I bring every decision and situation in my job to his attention. But his partnership with me extends to the work place, and I fit my roles into that framework.

Such flexibility, I have discovered, eases the burden of the partner who has extra demands on his time and energy.

## 2. Agree on Who Will Fill What Role

One should use common sense in dividing up household duties. I think this is harder for us men.

Many husbands do a few household chores and let their wives worry about the rest. They are insensitive to the heavy responsibility she carries in running the home smoothly.

Designate responsibilities for the home. Divide areas of management rather than assigning chores. Be creative. If your wife is an accountant and is willing, let her handle the finances. If your husband leaves for work an hour later than you do, ask him to make the beds and clear the breakfast dishes.

## 3. Use Humor to Ease the Strain

Once, during a trip to South Africa, I saw a full-page

ad listing men's winter suits for half price. The rand had devalued so I could buy clothes for 25 cents on the dollar. *What a bargain! Just in time for cool weather back home,* I reasoned.

So I bought four attractive suits for $90 each. In the United States, they would have cost $450 each, which is far more than I would have paid for a suit.

When I returned, however, I discovered that Vonette was far less excited about my purchases than I.

The minute I saw those suits, I didn't like them. I knew Bill was proud of the bargain he had made. But they were a different cut and looked frumpy on him. The coats were looser and longer than the suits he usually wears. And of course, the ugliest one of the batch was his favorite.

We agree on most things, but not on this one. When Bill appears in public, I want him to look his best. And I don't think he looks good in any of those suits.

When he starts to wear one of them, I gently remind him that he has something better-looking in his closet. But he just smiles at me and chuckles, "Every time I wear this suit is a day of ecstasy."

Those suits have become a joke between us. But underneath the banter, Vonette knows I respect her good taste in fashion.

We could have let a situation like this create tension between us. But, we laugh and chuckle and let our humor diffuse any differences of opinion.

## 4. Make Sure Your Roles Obtain the Desired Result

Many professional people tend to give their roles precedence over their partnership.

Zac's wife, Terry, has worked out her responsibility to her family with unusual perception. At one time, she had a job in which she was up for a promotion. Her company wanted her to be a district manager. Zac was attending seminary full-time and she needed to work.

But as a district manager, she would have to travel. This meant she would have to hire someone to care for their small children. Rebecca had spent much of her first six years in day care centers; Terry desired to be home more with baby Christopher than her current job would permit.

Realizing this new opportunity for advancing in the business would not give her enough time with the children and her husband, she refused the promotion and resigned from her job, giving up a very attractive salary. Now she cleans houses to supplement their income. Even though her new work is much harder and less prestigious, she can more adequately meet the needs of her husband and children. Her choice was not understood by her colleagues, but she finds her new role more fulfilling.

Keep your perspective clear. No position is so important that it should take precedence over your partnership. No job or career is successful if it leads to dissension or divorce. No expectation is so vital that you can let it fragment your family. Your roles do not merely maintain order in your home; they help you build closeness and unity in your relationship.

Vonette and I try to give God the liberty to be original in each other's lives. Walking together in spite of different expectations demonstrates commitment to partnership. Talk over your expectations. In so doing, you will understand your mate better and find more ways to complement him and help him achieve his goals. And in the process, you will learn to manage the changes you will surely encounter in the future.

## For Reflection, Discussion and Action

1. What expectations do you have of your spouse? Write them down. Now, how do they affect your partnership?

2. Name a specific situation which occurred recently where you could have minimized your stress by keeping roles flexible. How did you respond? How could you handle a similar situation better in the future?

3. How have you and your mate used humor to reduce tension? Do you need to utilize humor more often?

# 5

# *The Stress of Personality Differences*

Have you ever watched what happens when a dog unexpectedly crosses the path of a cat?

The dog stops dead in his tracks. The hair rises on his neck. His senses poise for battle.

The cat stiffens her tail. She arches her back. She extends her razor-sharp claws. She glares at him with yellow eyes.

A growl begins to rumble in his throat. She hisses and spits. Suddenly, he lunges at her. She slashes at his nose with lightning speed. They both back off, teeth bared. Growling. Hissing.

Some marriage conflicts can resemble this scene. When partners do not understand each other's differences, they disagree and argue. Sometimes they even "fight like cats and dogs."

Bill and I have very different personalities. He's intuitive and has amazing insights about people. I'm more analytical and try to make sure two plus two equals four.

He sees the broad scope of things; I notice the details. He always has time for people; I'm more time-conscious and task oriented. When I concentrate on projects, I sometimes lose sight of those around me.

Vonette is outgoing and enthusiastic. Although task oriented, she loves people, crowds and parties. She's hospitable and likes to open our home to guests. She's adept at making others feel comfortable. When she walks into a room, everyone responds to her warmth and humor.

I'm more reserved. While she can hold a conversation with eight people at a time, I feel more comfortable one-on-one.

And although I enjoy being with people, I prefer privacy. I would rather spend time with my wife, our children, or a few close friends than be involved with large crowds.

I'm a perfectionist and want to deal with things right away. Bill, sometimes out of necessity because of his schedule and responsibilities, has to live with ambiguity, loose ends and unfinished business.

I like color, convenience, pleasure, the "good life."

So sometimes I tell Vonette she's carnal. Then she gives me a wry smile.

Unlike Bill, I like things soft and gentle. I want people to treat me tenderly.

And when I remind her that I always treat her that way, she gives me that knowing look.

Over the years, our differences have bonded us together. If our personalities were the same, we would have a boring relationship. Vonette has brought sparkle to my life. Her zest and energy and appreciation of things I usually don't see has added much color to our marriage.

## Our Uniqueness

The character traits that make up a personality are so complex and intricate that no two persons are alike. Each of us has unique emotional and psychological attributes as well as distinctive physical characteristics.

If that isn't enough to make us one-of-a-kind, each personality also has been modified by a kaleidoscope of influences. Childhood training, education, past relationships, culture, background—all help to form one's character.

Our personality traits color and flavor our values—those things we consider important in life. In marriage, our values may clash.

For example, Bill and I value our possessions differently. I'm more materialistic than he. Sometimes I remind him that he enjoys much of what we have because I pray for it!

Years ago, about the time air conditioning in cars was becoming popular, we had to make a trip across country for staff training. Since we did not yet have air conditioning, we rigged up a system to make traveling through the desert tolerable. We set a large pan of ice on the floorboard of the passenger's side so the air from the vent would flow over the melting ice and cool the interior. As we drove, I wet towels in the cold water and hung them around the inside of the car for further cooling.

Proudly, we commented on how fortunate we were to

be riding in our comfortable "air conditioned" automobile. As cars passed us with windows rolled down, we felt sorry for the people who were sweltering in the heat.

I don't know how far we traveled like this, but we soon realized that those people weren't miserable after all. It had rained earlier, and the outside air was considerably cooler than the air inside our car.

Immediately, Bill stopped and we dumped our ice.

"This is it!" I exclaimed. "I am *not* making another trip without air conditioning."

Bill objected firmly. "Vonette, we can't have air conditioning when our staff members don't. It would be a poor example on our part."

"But they don't have the responsibilities and pressures on them that you do," I argued. "And many of them don't spend nearly as much time traveling either."

But he was adamant.

When we arrived at the conference, I noticed several of our staff driving air conditioned vehicles. So over the next year I prayed, "Lord, give us air conditioning if You please." And God graciously answered my prayer.

When we consider something important that our spouse doesn't, this can cause strain in our relationship. Some value differences are easy to resolve. Others are not.

One of the stresses of our marriage is how we each value Christmas presents. I love to see our Christmas tree piled with gifts. I would stack them to the ceiling because, to me, Christmas—as the celebration of our Lord's birthday—is one of the best times to show our love for the Lord and to each other through giving.

I disagree with Vonette.

There are so many other occasions, like birthdays and

anniversaries, when we can give to each other. I feel it is an insult to our Lord to spend lavishly on our family and friends at Christmastime. Don't get me wrong. Christmas is my favorite time of the year. I love the carols, the decorations and the tree. I just believe that all we do should glorify our Lord whose birthday we celebrate. I would much rather give to a charitable organization or to individuals in need in the name of our Lord than heap gifts on ourselves and our friends.

We could easily let our differences about Christmas gifts affect our partnership. We could destroy our togetherness during special times at Christmas by insisting on our own way. But Bill and I have worked out a happy compromise. And it has taken time and commitment from both of us to make it succeed.

We don't spend a lot on each other for presents; most of our giving goes to someone in need. But I make sure that our children and grandchildren are cared for, and I decorate the house and wrap the presents beautifully to heighten the festivity.

To build harmony in a relationship, we must recognize and accept our partner's values. Often this takes a lot of work, but the rewards are great.

## Managing Personality Differences

Some spouses seem to know instinctively how to generate marital harmony. They understand how to adapt to their mate's personality and reconcile their differences. Many couples, however, resort to destructive methods. They nag, suffer in silence, browbeat their partner.

Let's look at some practical ways we can handle personality differences positively, without losing our individual identities.

## 1. Understand Your Partner's Characteristics

The basis for handling the stress of personality differences is to thoroughly understand and accept your partner's characteristics. Even though understanding your differences won't solve every irritation and conflict, it will enable you to accept your partner.

By this we mean regard, value and highly esteem your mate. Understand that he acts differently because he *is* different. Don't try to change him. Instead, thank the Lord for giving you your spouse. Focus on his positive qualities. Develop a thankful spirit over each dissimilarity you find. Remember that Christ accepted you unconditionally and treat your partner in the same way.

## 2. Build Bridges Between Dissimilarities

The apostle Paul encourages us to "Pursue the things which make for peace and the building up of one another."[1] When our values don't match, it is easy to damage the special intimacy in our coupleness. Our task, then, is to build bridges between our differences.

Dissimilarities need not drive us apart. Actually, opposites attract, as you and your spouse may have discovered. We can use our unlikenesses to complement each other.

Bill and I function as a team. One day, we were running right on the minute and had an important appointment for which we didn't want to be late. As we hurried from Bill's office, a staff member with a serious personal problem met us.

"Bill! I need to talk to you . . . right away!"

"My dear friend, how may I help you?" Bill said warmly and ushered him into his office.

Bill has a compassionate heart for people and their needs. I tend to get caught up in tasks. Making appointments on time is a priority to me. He rounds out my personality in that area. If I had insisted on my way in that situation, we would have missed an opportunity for ministry and blessing.

Our intense loyalty to each other helps us build our bridges. God's Word says, "If you love someone, you'll be loyal to him no matter what the cost. You will always believe in him, always expect the best of him, and always stand your ground in defending him."[2] We see shortcomings in one another that no one else notices. But we talk about our weaknesses. We pray about them (in private). We care so much that we want to shield each other from hurt or humiliation. Because we have worked hard at building bridges between our dissimilarities, we are able to emerge from our private moments in unity.

### 3. Communicate

Lack of communication is one of the most common problems couples face in building bridges. Instead of talking out their differences, many spouses remain silent or resort to nagging.

Sometimes Vonette is tempted to nag me in situations where I have been negligent. I respond to her in one of two ways: Frequently I laugh at the situation and put my arms around her, telling her how beautiful she is and how much I love her. At first, this irritates her. But soon she's laughing with me, and the tension is over. Other times I lovingly remind her, "Now, look, your attitude is wrong. What are you going to do about it?" And I drop the subject. The next time we discuss it, things are all right.

I am grateful that she is honest with me in the same way.

Through communication, we can review our likes and dislikes and come up with God-given solutions. We can ask God to help us find answers to our disagreements.

## 4. Be Willing to Change

Communication often leads to change. But at what point should we expect our partner to change and when should we accept his differences?

There is no simple answer. Much depends on each spouse's need and the seriousness of the situation. Change may be necessary to build and maintain a harmonious relationship. Yielding to God's will also may require change.

I remember one occasion when I had to change. By nature, I'm cautious about making big moves. When Bill first showed me the hotel at Arrowhead Springs, I went into a tailspin.

Bill was convinced that Arrowhead Springs would help to accelerate our worldwide ministry in a dramatic way as a training center.

"What do we know about buying a hotel?" I objected. "What do we know about operating it? Why should we take on this huge responsibility?" The whole idea seemed overwhelming to me.

As we walked through the lobby and into one of the large meeting rooms, I noticed the worn carpet and tattered draperies. I imagined it would take a warehouse of paint to refurbish everything.

"We'll make the move by fall," Bill announced.

It was already July.

"Honey, you have to be crazy!" I protested. "We can't redo everything in that time."

But Bill was sure God wanted Campus Crusade to occupy Arrowhead Springs by fall.

I loved Bel Air where we lived. We were located three minutes from the heart of the UCLA campus, and hundreds of students had received Christ through our ministry there. Zac was settled in school and Brad loved nursery school. And I didn't want to leave Dr. Henrietta Mears with whom we had shared a home for ten years. I wanted other people to operate Arrowhead Springs while I stayed in my secure nest.

By the second of December, God had miraculously answered Bill's prayers and all of our offices had moved from Los Angeles to the hotel. Bill decided to live in the hotel, and I could come up on weekends. But I soon realized the impossibilities of this arrangement. Arrowhead Springs was to be a permanent part of our lives and ministry. I would have to make the change.

As I look back, I see how much the move meant to Bill and to the remarkable growth of Campus Crusade. He was confident of the Holy Spirit's leading. Had I refused to make the move, I would have caused serious problems in our relationship and hindered God's work.

We cannot always expect our spouse to change, however. It takes two to make harmony. There are some traits in our partners we must learn to accept. When one partner "gives in" all the time, resentment builds and communication breaks down. Decide how important your partner's needs and desires are and make your decisions accordingly.

## 5. Compromise

I value Vonette's opinions. She understands me better than anyone else, and she has a good mind and a loving heart. Her insights and wisdom help me make sound decisions. That is part of the beauty of our partnership.

Sometimes, however, we simply don't agree. No amount of talking will bridge the gap between our views. Then we have to compromise.

When each of us gives a little, we meet in the middle. And we try to guard against slighting our partner's deep-felt needs.

One morning Vonette and I got up early because we had a lot of work to do, and we had an early appointment at my office. We were praying together and meditating upon the Lord when suddenly we realized time had gotten away from us, and we were almost late for our appointment.

As we started to leave the house, Vonette noticed that our bed hadn't been made.

"Do that later, Vonette," I urged. "We shouldn't keep them waiting."

"But, Bill, we have guests coming for dinner, and I won't have time to come back and make the bed."

We debated for thirty seconds on what was more important, then took about four minutes to straighten the bedroom.

In our hurry to get out the door, I forgot to turn off the security alarm. Of course, our exit set it blaring. While I ran to reset it, Vonette slipped back in to arrange the pillows on the bed and make sure the laundry had been put in the basket. We were a few minutes late, but our compromise took some of the pressure off Vonette that evening.

## Using Differences to Strengthen Marriage

Strong marriages are built on divergent personalities. You will find that you can use your individuality to build channels of communication, to understand your partner, to develop sensitivity and compassion. Build your relationship on these qualities, and you will turn your marital differences into marriage strengtheners.

Think of the joy you felt when you were dating and began to discover the contributions your mate could bring to your marriage. Those strengths are still there. And those personality differences will bring balance to your oneness and keep your relationship from falling into a rut.

When you honestly confront your differences, you begin the process of fitting together. God created your mate to complement your personality and gifts, to strengthen your weaknesses and vulnerabilities. And you were made to do the same for him. Fitting together forges this unity.

We urge you to yield your disappointments and irritations to the Lord and apply these principles to your marriage. Building bridges with your mate is a lifetime of adventure and discovery.

## For Reflection, Discussion and Action

1. List what you see as your partner's personality characteristics and note how they differ from yours. Ask God to help you understand those characteristics and utilize this understanding in a positive way in your marriage.

2. Thank God for the qualities in your partner that you enjoy. Ask God to help you accept your partner unconditionally in the Spirit of Christ.

3. Discuss your dissimilarities with your partner. How can the two of you work together to build bridges between your differences and function as a team?

# 6

# *The Stress of Being an Entrepreneur*

If you have ever organized a special event, business venture or community project, you know first-hand that such endeavors rarely go smoothly. Disagreements, logistical problems and added responsibilities can add significant strain to your life, and possibly to your marriage.

Looking back over almost forty years of this ministry, I often marvel at the miracle of God's faithfulness to maintain a spirit of harmony and unity among the staff, especially the leadership. Not that there haven't been many opportunities for disagreements and misunderstandings.

You can imagine the potential for conflict with thousands of full-time and associate staff coming from many different backgrounds and cultures. And the stress that confrontations create can be enormous.

We faced a particularly stressful situation in preparing for Explo '72. We felt God wanted us to bring a great gathering of people to Dallas for a week of intensive training in discipleship and evangelism, which we envisioned would involve approximately 100,000 high school and college students, pastors and laypeople.

This was something Campus Crusade had never done. So my proposal was not met with a lot of excitement and enthusiasm. Some of the staff complained, "This will interfere with our ministry." From my perspective, I thought it would dramatically accelerate everything we were doing.

Although I felt strongly impressed of God that we should move ahead with plans for this event, I brought it before all our leadership so they would feel some ownership in it. Many of them didn't think the concept was a good idea nor did they believe it was of God. I encouraged our leaders to pray and talk further about the matter. Weeks passed and the opposition continued.

Finally, after six months of interaction and prayer, we called a meeting of our top leadership and vowed not to adjourn until the Lord had shown us clearly whether He wanted us to have the conference. After hours of prayer and discussion, the leaders were unanimously in favor. Later, however, some of the individuals who had previously opposed the event continued to sow discord.

At a subsequent meeting in Dallas, the majority of Campus Crusade's executive and middle management believed that we should go ahead with plans for the conference. Those who opposed continued to believe that their ministries would be sabotaged by the event, and some later resigned from Campus Crusade as a result.

That Dallas meeting was characterized by a spirit of repentance as we sought the will of the Lord together, and God blessed our decision to move ahead in a phenomenal way. Explo '72 became the greatest event up to that time in the history of the movement. The emphasis of the week was taken back to thousands of communities and churches from which those who attended had come. What Satan had tried to thwart, God turned into a great new era of ministry growth for Campus Crusade.

Dr. Joon Gon Kim, our director in Korea, experienced similar opposition to his proposal for Explo '74. Some of the Korean staff gave seventy-two reasons the conference couldn't happen. But Dr. Kim held fast to his conviction that God was leading him in this event and assured them of my support internationally. Several of the staff who objected resigned.

Explo '74 again proved to be the greatest event of its kind in our history. Night after night crowds ranged from 500,000 to 1½ million. One night, more than a million indicated salvation decisions for Christ. Millions more have been introduced to Christ through the hundreds of thousands who were trained at Explo '74.

In addition to knowing that there are thousands of other leaders who are committed to the vision which has guided Campus Crusade all these years, the one major factor that helps me deal with the stress of entrepreneurship is having Vonette by my side.

## Living As Entrepreneurs

From the beginning, we have been more interested in building disciples than in promoting our personal objectives. We believe that you cannot put people in boxes and make them dance to your tune. You must give them freedom within certain guidelines to follow the Holy Spirit's leading. Through the years we have helped train thousands of choice men and women for positions of leadership. One of our greatest joys has been been watching staff and students grow and develop as they are trained and given major responsibilities.

For the first fifteen years of this Campus Crusade for Christ ministry, I made all the major decisions with Vonette's help and counsel. I managed the organization, raised the funds, and was deeply involved in the ministry of evangelism and discipleship. All the time I prayed, "Lord, send me qualified help for these management responsibilities." But the burdens of running the organization only increased and our centralized leadership became cumbersome.

Finally, I concluded that Campus Crusade would cease to expand and be effective if it had to depend on one person for all its major activities. I simply would not be able to handle the stress of such a leadership-centered approach.

I began delegating more responsibility to various ministry heads. With the passing of time, their centers of activity were focused in other parts of the country. When they asked to relocate their offices, I agreed. Slowly, a system of management evolved that gave these leaders much freedom and authority to manage their affairs independently while staying within the overall objectives of Campus Crusade. Not even the danger of more challenges to my leadership would convince me to change this approach. I believe that potential leaders need room to grow and exercise their freedom and authority with responsibility and accountability.

Our organization continued to grow under this new format until today we have more than forty separate ministries with approximately 16,000 full-time and associate staff in all major countries around the world. Each ministry complements the others in helping to reach the world for Christ.

Even with the decentralization, however, the buck stops at my door. As the president and chief executive officer, I am ultimately accountable to the Lord to see that Campus Crusade accomplishes its goal of helping fulfill the Great Commission in the most Spirit-filled and productive manner. Keeping the various outreaches coordinated and working in the same direction is a challenge. But God has graciously given us the most able, gifted and godly leaders, we think, in the world.

Even so, you might imagine some of the stresses that Vonette and I face. The pressures of leading such a diverse organization, with an ever-growing financial budget, are tremendous. From a human standpoint, our lives should be a shambles. Indeed, apart from the grace of God and the power of the Holy Spirit, our marriage could not easily survive the strain.

We have to work at our relationship. By walking in the Spirit day-by-day, we have found that God enables us to remain faithful to our commitment to partnership and to helping fulfill the Great Commission.

My objective in our ministry is to complement Bill's leadership. In the early days, I worked with sorority women and other female students. Then when Bill started traveling, I filled in for him wherever I could.

We developed methods to train new Christians in how to set up a Bible study, how to contact students on campus, and how to schedule a sorority or fraternity house meeting.Finally, Bill decided to train college graduates by taking them witnessing on different campuses. We began to teach these willing workers right on the spot. Gradually, new training materials began taking shape. Working with the staff, I helped write many of the materials using the research I had done toward my master's thesis at USC.

After our headquarters moved to Arrowhead Springs in 1962, my role as a leader began to change. Our children, the beginning of the Lay Ministry, decorating the hotel, and training conferences consumed much of my time. Eventually, others brought their expertise to the staff and began making important decisions without my involvement.

As Explo '72 approached, I realized how little input I

had had in planning the event. The whole outreach was planned while I was on the sidelines.

The tremendous potential for this project thrilled me but I felt frustrated at being left out. "Lord," I complained, "this is the first time that I haven't been vitally involved in major decision making. I'm losing my influence in everything Bill and I have built together."

But God had a hand in this.

Earlier, I had met with Ruth Graham, Millie Dienert and Marion Lindsell. Millie shared with us how women in London had been organized into hundreds of prayer groups for one of Billy Graham's crusades. As we discussed the moral condition of our country, we agreed that the best way to make a significant impact in our own country was through prayer.

During my personal devotions, I came across Acts 4:24: "And the believers were united together in prayer." Suddenly, my thoughts clicked. *This is it! Prayer mobilization can unite Christians against the forces of evil in our land. With prayer, we can draw God's power into all the affairs of our nation.*

I called Bill. "Listen to the idea the Lord gave me!"

He was as excited as I was. "Outline your proposal and let's present it to the leadership," he suggested.

So I sat down and the ideas flowed from my pen. Within fifteen minutes, I had my strategy.

I brought it to Bill. He took one look at what I had written and exclaimed, "I like it. Do it!"

Bill and several other staff were leaving for Singapore to meet with our worldwide leadership. While he was gone, I went into action. All my plans fell easily into place. By the time he returned, meetings with prayer coordinators in six surrounding cities had taken place and a rally was planned for the Los Angeles Sports Arena with Ruth Graham as speaker.

When Bill heard of my activities, he mentioned that Explo '72 needed urgent prayer. So began the organizing of people into prayer groups and the mailing of prayer concerns.

With Bill's encouragement, the Great Commission Prayer Crusade was born, which became an arm of Campus Crusade. We helped conduct prayer workshops in churches, organized public prayer rallies, and mobilized people all over the United States to pray both inside and outside our ministry.

As this united force of prayer caught on, my personal ministry expanded. The National Prayer Committee developed out of many prayer efforts springing up all over the country. Eventually, the committee took on the responsibility for promoting the National Day of Prayer for which I have had the privilege of being chairman for several years.

In 1974 the Lausanne Committee for World Evangelization, an outgrowth of the Billy Graham ministry, was formed. I became a part of the Intercession Working Group and in 1979 accepted the challenge to chair that group. This included serving on the Executive Committee of the LCWE.

In 1984 the LCWE and the Korean Evangelical Fellowship sponsored the International Prayer Assembly where people from seventy countries gathered in Seoul, Korea. This was a dream come true as the meeting sparked prayer movements all over the world. It was a great privilege to co-chair that tremendous event.

Involvement in a prayer ministry has added to our entrepreneurial responsibilities. The tensions of our work could easily separate us. But our commitment to partnership has given us the platform from which to work through the pressures.

## Stressors of Entrepreneurship

Handling crises in leadership is not my only source of stress as an entrepreneur. I have the responsibility of giving leadership to New Life 2000,* the largest and most comprehensive strategy for world evangelization our ministry has ever undertaken. That effort is constantly before me.

Vonette and I also care deeply for our staff and their problems. We spend time counseling those in financial crisis or facing sickness and the loss of loved ones.

Many ministry leaders need ten or fifteen minutes or an hour of my day. Telephone calls, dictation, articles I need to write, correspondence, urgent interruptions, and co-authoring this book are my other current stressors.

My daily schedule and extensive travel cause strain. I often spend more hours flying than sleeping in my own bed. I take manuscripts or unanswered correspondence with me on trips so I can work on the plane or in my hotel room. As I travel, I look for someone with whom to share Christ. And though I've traveled for many hours, I have to appear refreshed as I disembark. Oftentimes my hosts forget about jet lag and missed rest and expect me to speak as soon as I get off the plane. And I always want to be prepared.

Managing all these stressors effectively is essential to preserving my marriage and family life. "To whom much

---

\* New Life 2000 is the registered service mark of Campus Crusade for Christ, Inc. New Life 2000 is a movement sponsored by Campus Crusade working in cooperation with millions of Christians in thousands of churches of most denominations and hundreds of mission groups. We are in the process of raising one billion dollars to establish 5,000 New Life Training Centers and 10,000 "JESUS" film teams. Our objective is to help present the gospel to more than six billion people by the year 2000, to introduce one billion to Christ, and plant one million new churches.

is given, much is required." We share our commitments not in pride or so you will feel sorry for us, but to help you see that it is possible to cope no matter what the circumstances.

While I share many of Bill's pressures, I have some stressors of my own: Raising funds and having enough staff to coordinate the National Day of Prayer. Depending on other people and finding that they don't always follow through. Interpersonal relationships. Training new staff. Managing the details of the office and home. And trying to keep up with Bill.

We would not want to wish our lifestyle on anyone else. This is what we have chosen to do as an expression of our love for Christ and our desire to obey Him. We are blessed with energy and good health, and both of us are born activists.

But stress is not unique to entrepreneurs. Countless couples live on the fast track. Ministers, business executives, and two-career couples all face similar pressures.

Let's look at some of the stressors they endure.

## 1. Overwork

Success and work can become addictive. Vonette and I have seen many couples grow apart because one partner couldn't keep his work in perspective.

If your career is breaking up your relationship, give it up. If you have a problem with overwork, set stringent limits on yourself.

Your partner is the most important person in your life. If you put your career before your spouse, you may make bushels of money but be miserable in the process. Ultimately, the only thing that really matters is your relationships with the Lord, your life partner and your family.

## 2. Family Activities Out of Balance

In this ministry we have always placed a strong emphasis on the importance of family. We have encouraged fathers and mothers to be lovingly involved in the various activities of their children. At the same time we recognize that some parents in today's society are so concerned about their children that they don't give proper attention to their profession. They spend an inordinate amount of time attending athletic events, PTA meetings and social functions. When kept in balance, these activities are valuable for the family. But when they begin to infringe on job or ministry responsibilities, they can be detrimental.

At times husbands demand too much time from their wives, and wives from their husbands. Not that spending time with your family is wrong. Sometimes, however, family concerns can consume too much of our time and energy. To establish a proper balance, husband and wife need to constantly re-evaluate and reaffirm their priorities to the Lord and to each other.

## 3. Independent Spirit

When both husband and wife have responsible career positions, they frequently develop independent lifestyles. The deadly factor is that this independence develops so gradually and subtly that the couple is unaware of it.

The U.S. Bureau of Labor Statistics reports that 17 percent of men and 10 percent of women in the work force do not work the traditional 8-to-5 shift. And the trend is expected to continue.[1] As a result, many dual career couples spend more time apart than together.

Because of schedule conflicts, they attend social functions separately, have less opportunity to support each other and share less physical and emotional contact. Soon they slip into patterns of independent living.

She joins a spa; he takes up tennis. She spends her Saturday working for a charity; he goes on a fishing trip. Both are so busy climbing separate corporate ladders that they rarely pay attention to each other. Living in a divided house, their partnership dissolves like warming Jell-O.

Is your marriage suffering from the stress of self-reliance? It takes planning and commitment to overcome the handicaps of living separate lives. Make a point to include each other in decision-making. Schedule time together; don't expect it to "just happen." Use the telephone to keep in contact.

**4. Women as professionals**

Many women involved in high-level careers find new strains in their marital relationships. Bill and I have observed couples who have separated because their working roles destroyed their partnership.

I would encourage a professional wife to stay alert to her husband's response to her career. If their working roles contribute to an improper relationship at home, they should set definite guidelines for their partnership and continuously evaluate their responses and needs. If they find their togetherness eroding, they should immediately remedy the problem—if necessary by changing careers.

## Principles for Reducing the Stress

Vonette and I have discovered two principles that have enabled us to reduce our stress as entrepreneurs: loving by faith and good stewardship of our time, talent and treasure.

During the height of one time of crisis and stress, the Lord revealed to me one of the most important truths I've ever taught—how to love by faith.* Early one morning I

---

\* For further information on how to love by faith, see *Transferable Concepts for Powerful Living* (Here's Life Publishers).

was awakened from a deep sleep. I felt impressed to get up, open my Bible, and kneel to read and pray. What I discovered during the next two hours has since enriched my life and the lives of countless others.

Briefly, the concept is this: We love by faith. Everything about the Christian life is based on faith. We love by faith just as we received Christ by faith and just as we are filled with the Holy Spirit by faith.

Jesus has *commanded* us to "love each other as much as I love You."[2] God *promises* that if we ask anything according to His will, He hears and answers us.[3] Relating this promise to God's command, we can claim by faith the privilege of loving with His love.

When I began to practice loving by faith, I found that conflicts with other individuals seemed to disappear, often miraculously.

Loving by faith has enabled me to continue loving those who through the years have sought to hinder God's vision for this ministry. To this day, if I were to meet any one of them on the street, I would be able to give each a warm embrace and truthfully say, "I love you."

Vonette and I also have discovered that good stewardship of our time, talent and treasure is foundational for handling the stressors of entrepreneurship or a dual career. The whole of life — our personality, influence, material substance, and especially our family — is His. He holds us accountable for what He has given us.[4]

We encourage you to dedicate all your resources — your time and talents as well as your treasure — to the lordship of Jesus Christ. Commit yourself to prayer and God's Word. Make fellowship with the Lord the center of your day. Walk with Him and talk with Him continuously. Your trust in God will help you put into perspective the demands and strains you face.

Invest in your personal wholeness as well. Reserve time for family and friends outside your workplace. Discover your chief interests and incorporate them into your work and leisure hours. If you realize the creative potential in your life, you will keep daily pressures manageable.

We have discovered that the stability and support of a loving marital relationship provides the platform of freedom and security you need to launch and maintain your career.

Build on your partnership and watch how your oneness adds to your abilities at work. Find the security and comfort of having that one special person who will help you develop your talents and share your successes for a lifetime.

## For Reflection, Discussion and Action

1. Do either you or your spouse function in the role of an entrepreneur? How does this situation affect your marriage relationship?

2. This week, at the end of each day, jot down in a notebook the number of hours that you spent: (a) doing work-related tasks, (b) being with your children, (c) being exclusively with your spouse, and (d) praying and meditating on God's Word. Will you adjust your schedule for next week? How?

# 7

# *The Stress of Divided Loyalties*

Perhaps you have discovered as Bill and I have that the demands from ministry, career, family, neighbors and friends can sometimes be overwhelming. The obligations seem to stack like gridlock on a freeway. Schedules fall into disarray, causing conflicts, stress and guilt. At such times it is easy to feel pulled apart by conflicting loyalties.

I recall an incident when we lived in Bel Air with Henrietta Mears . . .

Brad was in his high chair. He loved to curl his tongue and let dribbles of cereal run out the corners of his mouth. Five-year-old Zac had taken a glass milk bottle off the table and had been pushing it along the lines of the kitchen floor tiles while simulating the sounds of a truck. Finding the metal legs of the high chair, he began to bump it and honk. This irritated Brad, who started to cry.

Just then the telephone rang. I ignored it at first, hoping Miss Mears would get it in another room. But she didn't. I had to abandon the brewing storm in the kitchen to answer it.

Bill was phoning long distance. He had been traveling for some weeks speaking and interviewing potential staff. Grabbing a pencil, I wrote down his new flight arrival schedule into Los Angeles.

Zac was still banging into the high chair and Brad was still crying when I returned. I glanced at the kitchen counter and sink. Twenty-five glass cups and plates from last night's student gathering still waited to be washed. A bowl of cookie dough with only half the ingredients sifted into it demanded my attention. Miss Mears had requested them for an afternoon tea for Sunday school teachers, but the boys had awakened before I could complete the mixture. It wasn't even 8 A.M., and I felt exhausted.

I moved Zac's milk bottle around the high chair leg and began washing the oatmeal off Brad's face and neck.

In reality, motherhood didn't resemble the colorful magazine ads for Carter's layette. It felt more like the center ring under a circus big top. On either side were arenas that demanded Vonette Zachary Bright's performance. One was the ministry; another, motherhood; another, my relationship with Bill. Then there were the tasks of the house and Miss Mears. Any of them alone could have filled my time. I was the performer who did juggling acts, balanced on high wires, and jumped through hoops of fire.

I sighed.

Miss Mears breezed into the kitchen carrying a tray strewn with the remains of her breakfast tea — toast crusts and a smudge of marmalade. She deposited it on the counter.

Her voice sang. "Good morning to you, dear. I thought I would finish my devotions in the garden."

Groomed in lovely summer cotton from her dressmaker, she had tucked an edition of *My Utmost for His Highest* under her arm. I felt the contrast in our appearance. I wore an old apricot colored robe that zipped up the front. It had random spots of baby cereal in its fleece, and the cuff was wet from contact with a wash cloth.

I identified with Martha in the Bible who was burdened with much serving while her sister Mary attended to the Lord. Like Martha, I resented the daily onslaught of demands.

Carrying Brad and towing Zac, I took the boys to our side of the house to get dressed. I would come back to the cookie dough and dishes.

On the way, I saw that the faded flowers in the dining room vases needed replacing. I told Zac to pick up his plastic boat between the legs of the formal chair. With my free arm, I gathered the one load of clean laundry left on the couch.

Once in the bedroom, I cried. I wasn't simply having a bad morning. It had been like this for months and I felt frustrated and depressed. *How can I do all this and keep up my end of the ministry, too?*

Glancing at the calendar on the desk, I looked forward to Bill's return. How I wished he knew how to slay some dragons . . .

High demands lead to dissatisfaction at work and at home, and can cause incredible emotional stress in a marriage. And resentment. Depression. Fatigue. Bitterness. All kinds of crises can erupt from the pressure of too many things to do.

No matter who feels the tension, it affects both partners. They may blame each other for the pressure they feel. They may develop rivalry in trying to resolve their conflicts.

Instead of achieving oneness, a couple under stress can find themselves strained and pulled apart.

## Dealing With Divided Loyalties

How do you handle your divided loyalties? Most couples manage theirs haphazardly. They respond to the "tyranny of the urgent" and ignore more important priorities. As a result, their lives become unbalanced. They feel guilty, and this provokes more conflict and uneasiness. Frustration builds and tempers flare. Let us share three suggestions that have helped us in dealing with this problem.

### 1. Maintain a Clear Perspective

If we are struggling under a cloud of condemnation, we cannot have a clear perspective on the demands on our life. Sometimes, for example, I think about all those boxes that need sorting in the basement and the bottom of our closets, or about all the little things in my office I should attend to. If I didn't recognize the low priority they have on my calendar and send them back to their rightful spot on the back burner, these insignificant details would drain my energy.

Those boxes in the closets do not bother me as they do Vonette. What does loom over me are my stacks of correspondence and neglected reading, and my constant deadlines on books, articles and sermons. It would be easy to feel guilty about not being able to meet all the expectations and demands of our ministry. But I try to keep things in perspective by reminding myself there is only so much I can do. So I do what I can, then try to relax. Although my days are long and meetings and conferences numerous, I have had to learn to cast my cares on the Lord, as we have been commanded to do.[1]

### 2. Build Bridges Through Partnership

Through partnership, we can blend the joys and stresses of our busy lifestyle to create a symphony of growth and pleasure. Even the sad, dark experiences will add significance to our marriage.

Building bridges through partnership will enable you to ease the pressure of expectations, meet your challenges day-by-day, work through your differences, and overcome the temptation to live independent lives.

The first task in this process is to define your loyalties and determine the priorities in your relationship. Understanding what is important and what has priority will give direction and consistency to your relationship and provide the foundation for whatever you do. From this platform you can evaluate the demands on you and formulate a plan to deal with them.

Bill and I have used the contract we signed with the Lord early in our marriage many times to enhance the bridges of our partnership and keep ourselves committed to the Lord and to each other. Our partnership requires that we work daily at achieving the things we agreed on.

Flexibility is essential to bridge building. As we write, San Francisco is slowly digging out from under the rubble of a deadly earthquake. Measuring 7.1 on the Richter scale, the fifteen-second temblor killed sixty-seven people and left thousands injured and homeless. Buildings, streets and bridges suffered more than seven billion dollars in damage—making it the costliest natural disaster in U.S. history.

Many commuters lost their lives when the top levels of the Oakland Bay Bridge and Nimitz Freeway collapsed onto the bottom lanes. But despite the structural failure of these and other bridges in the disaster area, the famous Golden Gate Bridge survived.

In this incident, the incredible ability of the bridge to

flex with the tremor saved the Golden Gate. Because its roadbed rests in a massive sling of cables and span that sway when rocked by a quake, the bridge weathered the catastrophe with little more than a superficial crack or two.

Flexing with the tremors of life will help you keep your marriage partnership undamaged when divided loyalties threaten disaster. Many good resources are available to help you in this process. You could attend one of the many fine marriage seminars sponsored by Campus Crusade's Family Ministry, for example. Your pastor or a professional Christian counselor also can help.

### 3. Cultivate a Thankful Attitude

An attitude of thankfulness also has helped Bill and me manage the stresses of divided loyalties.

One morning years ago I sat next to Bill, seething as he backed the car out of the driveway. How perfect we looked! The backdrop of our home was stately. As a family we were going to church. Zac and baby Brad were in sailor suits with knee socks. But I felt like a hypocrite. Outwardly the canvas was perfectly colored with correct forms, but on the back side were dark blotches of anger.

At breakfast I had tried to communicate to Bill my growing frustration over having to perform repetitive tasks. His response seemed so shallow. He called it "Spiritual Breathing," outlining how I should "exhale" a confession of my sin and "inhale" the power of the Holy Spirit by claiming God's promises by faith. I felt too out of control for such simplicity.

At church that morning I noted in the bulletin that the guest speaker's address was entitled "Looking Up." I sighed. *More weary platitudes that float above our heads.* I yearned for more substance than the allotted thirty minutes of lofty language. The speaker's opening remarks felt like a prophetic word:

Dissatisfaction and frustration are not of God. If we are dissatisfied about something, we should ask God what is causing us to be that way and then ask Him to remove it. If He doesn't remove it, we are to ask what He wants us to learn from that situation.

I felt deaf to any continuing speech. I had been praying to be out of the Moorish castle in which we lived, or for the aid of an efficient housekeeper. I clearly knew that the Lord had not allowed either. What was He trying to teach me? Deep inside, I didn't even know if I wanted to learn, whatever it was.

The Tuesday night College Life meetings in our home were drawing such enormous crowds that Bill and the staff had to push the living room and dining room furniture into auxiliary halls.

The terrible part was that I wanted to be out with the students, but I ended up spending most of the time in the kitchen preparing refreshments. It had always seemed like a mismanagement of talent; I could explain the steps to salvation with brevity and clarity, and I wanted to introduce these students to Christ. Yet, I mixed punch while younger staff members sometimes tripped in their presentation.

As I listened to the speaker, I held up my observation to God, and He provided me with clear insight. The young staff needed the experience for training. It was as if one sliver of discontent had been extracted, and the wound filled with balm.

I put my arm through Bill's. It was so clearly a battle of attitude and not circumstance. I made a decision that morning to give thanks in my situation and work on performing every task as unto the Lord.

I learned the practical application of 1 Thessalonians 5:18, "No matter what happens, always be thankful, for this is God's will for you who belong to Christ Jesus."[2] I began to thank God for the dishes, the diapers, the dust, the drudgery. The result was amazing. I began to find joy in the tasks that I had formerly resented. I experienced a new sense of victory and excitement in living for and serving Christ.

Perhaps you can think of a time in your life when giving thanks has quieted the storm of conflicting demands upon you. I have learned that, whenever I respond to conflict with a thankful attitude, the demands roaring at me are muzzled. Their voices diminish until I see them in perspective. Then I can sort them out and deal with them one by one.

We encourage you to maintain a clear perspective on the daily pressures of career, family and spiritual life. See yourself and your spouse as partners in life. Construct flexible bridges across the chasms of your differences. And ask the Holy Spirit to help you establish God-centered priorities for an intimate, joyful, Spirit-filled marriage.

By following these principles, and those we will share in the following pages, you will learn how to prevent or reduce many of the stresses in your relationship.

## For Reflection, Discussion and Action

1. A dual career produces divided loyalties. Describe the divided loyalties which you have experienced. What stress has this caused in your marriage?

2. How can partnership in marriage bridge divided loyalties?

3. Flexibility and compromise are effective tools for managing divided loyalties. Describe how you plan to use these tools to manage your marriage partnership.

# *Step 2*

## Establish God-Centered Priorities

*To ensure their partnership and help prevent many of the stresses in marriage, couples must establish God-centered priorities that reflect their values and help accomplish their goals.*

# 8

# *The Throne Check*

When the Crystal Palace Exhibition opened in 1851, people flocked to London's Hyde Park to view the marvels. Steam power had captured the imagination of inventors. Lines of people gaped at the steam plows, steam locomotives, steam looms, steam organs and even a steam cannon.

But first prize went to an exhibit that defied description. It boasted seven thousand moving parts. Its pulleys clanked, whistles shrieked, bells clanged and gears ground, all making an incredible noise. But the contraption didn't do a thing. In spite of the motion and commotion, the machine had no practical use.

Have you ever felt a little like that machine? Spinning countless plans, whirling through innumerable projects, and passing by the hours, but accomplishing little?

Sometimes it's easy to fool ourselves by mistaking action for achievement.

Perhaps you have experienced this in your marriage. Your relationship wins a blue ribbon in the eyes of others, but you realize that your goals and dreams are being shattered by frenzied activity. You frequently become sidetracked from doing what you and your spouse agree is best for your unity.

Vonette and I want to share some practical principles that we are convinced will bring purpose and great rewards to your marriage as they have ours: how you can build godly attitudes and establish God-centered priorities that will help prevent many of the stresses in your relationship.

## Choosing Attitudes

An attitude is a "mindset" that continuously influences how we view ourselves, our situations, other people and relationships. Attitude is a matter of the will. We have the power to choose how we think and react. Our mindset filters all the information we receive and colors our judgments and responses.

Godly attitudes build godly marriages. Like constructing an intricate machine, building a marriage is hard, delicate work. No one achieves it by accident. Our values and goals bring purpose to the mechanism. Our priorities form the internal works and gears that make it run. But the device will grind to a halt if we fail to provide one more ingredient—lubrication. In marriage, godly attitudes oil the flow of partnership so that it can function with a minimum of friction.

## Setting Priorities

Priorities are like roads on a well-marked map pointing the way to our destination. Stress comes when we stray from our course and follow patterns of behavior that balloon differences into major conflicts. Let's look at the Christian couple's roadmap for a moment.

The main thoroughfare is a *vital spiritual life.* This includes a dynamic, personal walk with our Savior and Lord

Jesus Christ, and a godly communion with your spouse. Surrendering to the lordship of Christ and living through the power of the Holy Spirit enables you to enjoy a Spirit-filled marriage.

The second major route on the map of priorities is *godly stewardship*. God has entrusted you with the resources you need for a successful marriage. By following biblical principles for stewardship, you will experience less friction in your relationship.

Sometimes along the way, however, you explore avenues which lead only to dead ends. Detours often slow couples down. But you must stay on the boulevards to succeed. In the following pages we will survey these roads carefully. Our journey begins with the "main thoroughfare."

## Vital Spiritual Life

Vonette and I find that to enjoy a strong and intimate partnership, we must put God first in our marriage. We must surrender absolutely to the lordship of Christ. We must yield totally to the control of the Holy Spirit.

Let me illustrate. I was speaking one evening to several hundred couples. As I stood behind the lectern, I noticed one particularly attractive couple sitting close to the front on my left. She held her head confidently, and had fine, classical features. His rough-hewn looks complemented hers.

After I finished my talk, this couple rushed up to me. When the crowd thinned, we sat together in a corner of the room.

"We're planning to get a divorce," the young man explained immediately.

His remark caught me by surprise. "Tell me a little about yourselves."

"We've been married two years and have worked in Christian ministry the entire time."

I looked at her. "That sounds like an exciting life. What's the problem?"

"I don't like my wife's looks," he blurted impatiently.

Surprised, I laughed. It was one of the most ridiculous statements he could have made.

"What are you laughing about?" he muttered, offended.

"Your wife is a beautiful woman. I can't imagine why you would say you don't like her appearance."

Apparently, that young husband was letting sinful thoughts ruin his love for his wife. Even though he wanted his marriage to succeed, his mindset was distorting their relationship.

I explained that every Christian has two natures: The Bible describes one as the "old man" or "the flesh." The other is called the "new man," representing the person who walks in the power of the Holy Spirit.

I took a sheet of paper and began drawing the following diagram:

**Our Control Center**

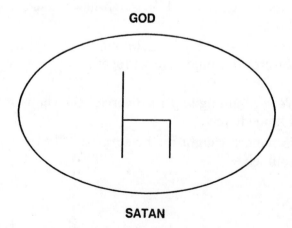

"This circle," I explained, "represents what I call the throne room in your life. The chair symbolizes a throne— the control center of your life. There are two spiritual kingdoms seeking to influence us. One is God's kingdom and the other is Satan's. Before we became Christians, as members of Satan's kingdom, we had no choice but to yield to his influence. But when we received Christ, we surrendered our 'control center' to Him."*

Then I added to the diagram:

**Freedom of Choice**

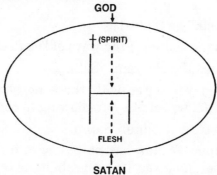

To explain the additions, I asked both of them to turn in their Bibles to Galatians 5:16,17. "Here," I pointed out, "the apostle Paul describes the ongoing conflict that takes place between the kingdom of God and the kingdom of Satan:

> I advise you to obey only the Holy Spirit's instructions. He will tell you where to go and what to do, and then you won't always be doing the wrong things your evil nature wants you to.
>
> For we naturally love to do evil things that are just

---

* For a more in-depth discussion of this principle, I encourage you to read my book, *The Secret: How to Live With Purpose and Power* (Here's Life Publishers).

the opposite from the things that the Holy Spirit tells us to do; and the good things we want to do when the Spirit has his way with us are just the opposite of our natural desires. These two forces within us are constantly fighting each other to win control over us, and our wishes are never free from their pressures (TLB).

"Our two natures, the spirit and the flesh, battle one another for our attention. God gives us freedom of choice, and we often allow the flesh to retake the throne."

I turned to the young man. "Which nature do you suppose is responsible for your critical attitude concerning your wife?"

"The flesh," he replied.

"Who is the source of the ways of the flesh?"

He studied the diagram. "Satan."

"So when you agree with those negative thoughts about your wife, whom are you allowing to control you?"

His face turned white. "Satan."

I continued. "Satan has no power to break up marriages. He does, however, have the ability to tempt and entice us with every kind of evil. We have the choice to say yes or no to his clever, subtle and devious temptations.

"When we as Christians live in sin, we are still in God's possession, but we have yielded to the influence of Satan and given the flesh control of the throne. Christ is no longer on the throne, but He continually seeks to influence us and bring us back to God's ways. As long as we allow our fleshly nature to remain on the throne, our attitudes and actions will be selfish and sinful."

I added a radio dial to the diagram:

## Making the Right Choice

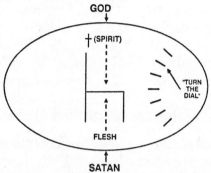

"We have the choice whether to listen to Satan's lies or to God," I explained. "We can consciously decide to 'turn the dial,' as on a radio, and listen to a better program— God's program! And God's program is to help you love your wife with your whole heart. What would you like to do?"

"Turn the dial," he said with a Cheshire grin.

So we bowed in prayer and committed his new attitude to the Lord.

When I happened to see the couple an hour later, he said, "She looks better to me already." He grinned and hugged her.

She smiled with pleasure.

Six months later, I was walking down the hallway of a building on a campus when I observed at a distance a couple swinging hands and looking at each other with adoring glances. Suddenly, we recognized each other. It was this same couple. They exclaimed over and over how much they appreciated my counsel at our previous meeting.

"We have been using that diagram which you shared with us to help other people with marital problems," he enthused.

"It also can be used in helping people with other problems," she chimed.

Through the years, I have used this diagram of the throne hundreds of times to explain almost every kind of temptation and conflict. And I have applied its life-changing truth to my own daily life. A daily "Throne Check," as I call it, is crucial to a vital spiritual life. It's what keeps Vonette and me on the road to marital success.

## Principles for a Spiritual Marriage

Bill has commented, "Because Vonette and I are both such strong personalities, it is not likely that we would be married today unless we were living Spirit-filled lives." I agree. I marvel that any couple who doesn't live for God in the power and control of the Holy Spirit can stay together in our stressful world.

The Lord understands the struggles we face in putting our trust in Him. He knows we cannot have faith on our own; it is a gift from Him.[1] That is why He sent His Holy Spirit to help us fight our battles.

He also has given many spiritual principles in His Word to help us build a Spirit-filled marriage. Bill shares five of these truths now.

### 1. Be in Love With the Lord

A love relationship with the Lord Jesus Christ is basic to establishing a spiritual marriage. Jesus said, "You shall love the Lord with all your heart, and with all your soul and with all your mind. This is the foremost commandment."[2]

God places a high premium on love. A careful study of Revelation 2 reveals that the church at Ephesus did many commendable things. It worked hard for the Lord; it didn't tolerate sin among its members; it was even willing to suffer for Christ. But God was displeased with the church because it had left its first love for Him.

Many Christians today are like this church. They busy

themselves day and night serving the Lord, but in the process they have left the first love that characterized their new life in Christ.

I'm often asked the question, "What is the most important thing you would like people to pray for you?" My answer is always the same: "That I may never leave my first love."

God desires our love just as we desire the love of our children. An incident that happened several years ago illustrates this: One evening I was at the table studying while Vonette worked in another part of the house. Zac, who was then in his early teens, came into the room carrying half a dozen books. Without interrupting me, he set them on the table and began reading quietly.

Suddenly, I became conscious of his presence beside me. "Son, is there something I can do for you?" I asked softly.

"No, Dad. I just want to be near you."

Imagine how I felt! His words melted my heart. He could have gone a hundred places to be alone with his books. But he chose to be with me. That's how our precious Savior feels when our gratitude and love for Him makes us ache to be with Him.

## 2. Read the Word of God

If we are in love with Jesus, we will want to read His Word daily. The Bible is His love message to us, and we will want to discover how to please Him more each day. The psalmist declares:

> Oh, the joys of those . . . [who] delight in doing everything God wants them to, and day and night are always meditating on his laws and thinking about ways to follow him more closely.
>
> They are like trees along a river bank bearing lus-

cious fruit each season without fail. Their leaves shall never wither, and all they do shall prosper.[3]

Like those trees, our spirits grow strong and healthy when we consistently read, study, memorize and meditate on God's Word. Sharing the Scriptures as a couple enables us to mature together in spiritual understanding and marital intimacy.

### 3. Spend Time in Prayer

No matter how much public ministry we have or how many individuals we introduce to Christ, that's only part of our lives. The success or failure of our marriage and our service to the Lord stems from the private sanctuary of our hearts. A consistent prayer life keeps us in touch with the Source of our success. No one knew this better than our Lord. He also taught His disciples to pray and abide in Him and His Word.[4] His example alone should convince us of the importance of prayer and meditation in building a solid relationship.

Vonette and I have learned how important it is to take time each day to be alone with God. Our marriage, as well as our ministry, depends on it. We cannot possibly live the life of a victorious, fruitful Christian without nourishing our spiritual natures *daily*.

Bill and I try to "pray without ceasing."[5] We want to fill our days with God's presence. We each have our private times alone with the Lord, though we also seek to enhance our relationship with each other by praying together. Whenever we are together, we begin and end each day on our knees for a brief time in prayer. Throughout the day we seek to maintain constant communication with our Lord. Prayer, meditating on His Word and listening to recorded hymns of worship and praise are part of our lifestyle. Many times during the day we lift our hearts in praise or silent prayer. Often we join members of our staff or other Christians in prayer.

We talk a lot about intimacy these days. How much closer can husbands and wives be than when they come united into God's presence? Through our years of praying together, we have learned to understand each other better; we care more and feel each other's pain and joy more fully.

Prayer enables us to place our stresses at the feet of Jesus. Often Bill and I hold hands as we pray about our differences. God becomes our loving arbitrator. Even when we differ on an issue, we can agree in prayer, "Lord, we need Your wisdom. Show us what's right. Help us to handle this situation for Your glory."

As we pray, we don't worry about saying fancy theological words. We simply express our love to God and to each other and ask Him to guide our steps. My heart feels especially warmed when Bill asks the Lord to "Walk around in my body, think with my mind, speak with my lips, love with my heart; and because Christ came to seek and to save those who are lost, I ask that you will seek and save the lost through me today." That is my prayer, too.

## 4. Live a Holy Life

Bill and I have discovered that walking close to the Lord and obeying His commands help us keep "short accounts" with God. The apostle Paul urges:

> As obedient children, do not be conformed to the former lusts which were yours in your ignorance, but like the Holy One who called you, be holy yourself in all your behavior; because it is written, "You shall be holy, for I am holy."[6]

How can Christians live holy lives? Through the years Bill has taught a concept he calls "Spiritual Breathing." Like physical breathing, Spiritual Breathing is a process of exhaling the impure and inhaling the pure. It is an exercise in faith that enables you to experience God's love and forgiveness as a way of life.

To keep "short accounts" in your spiritual life and in your marriage, you can breathe spiritually the moment the Holy Spirit convicts you of sin or shortcomings.

First, "exhale" by confessing that sin to God, for the Bible says that "If we confess our sins, He is faithful and just to forgive us our sins and to cleanse us from all unrighteousness."[7]

Confession in its original sense means to agree with God. Basically, there are three ways to agree with God: (1) that whatever you do that grieves the Holy Spirit is sin — pride, jealousy, lust, critical spirit; (2) Christ has paid the penalty by dying on the cross and shedding His blood for your sins; and (3) you repent; as an act of your will you agree to change your attitude toward your acts of disobedience, which results in a change of action. You begin to obey God instead of disobeying Him. One cannot be a victorious Christian and experience a meaningful marriage relationship if he has unconfessed sin in his life.

Next, "inhale" by receiving God's forgiveness and cleansing and by appropriating the fullness of the Holy Spirit in your life by faith.

God *commands* Christians to be filled with the Holy Spirit as a way of life.[8] He *promises* to hear and answer all our prayers that are consistent with His will.[9] Therefore, we can claim His fullness as an act of the will by faith based on His holy, inspired Word.

If done with a genuine desire to please God and achieve victory over sin in your life or marriage, Spiritual Breathing is all it takes to make things right between you and your heavenly Father. And it will enable the Holy Spirit to bless your marriage.

Bill and I place a strong emphasis on the role of the Holy Spirit in a happy marriage because every self-effort to find happiness is doomed to failure. Only the Holy Spirit can enable us to experience the happy, fulfilled marriage that God has ordained for His children.

## 5. Apply the Throne Check

Through the years, Bill and I have used the Throne Check to test our attitudes and actions. When one of us catches himself or another member of the family doing something that doesn't please God, we gently ask the question, "Who's on the throne?"

The Throne Check provides the theological basis for relationship in our family. It reminds us of our need to have our Lord Jesus Christ in control of our lives at all times. This simple device helps us to see that the person in the wrong is not the problem. The issue to consider is who is in control, the flesh or the Spirit? The Throne Check has enabled us to resolve many difficulties that could have erupted into major conflict.

We explained this concept to the boys one night when Zac was nine years old and Brad was five. Then we asked, "Zac, who's on the throne? Brad, who's on the throne?"

Both answered, "Jesus."

Lesson learned. Well, not quite.

The next morning at breakfast, I cooked a dish called "egg-in-a-bonnet." I had found the recipe somewhere and wanted to try it. I cut a hole in the middle of each slice of bread and fried it in butter on one side. Then I turned it over to toast on the other side, and placed a raw egg inside the hole, covering the skillet to let it cook. It made a pretty breakfast with the toasted round center of bread placed over the egg to look like a bonnet.

When Brad came to the table, he looked at his food and

turned up his nose. "I'm not going to eat it!" he exclaimed. "I don't want my egg that way."

We didn't take it too seriously because he had never acted like that before. The rest of us started eating. But Brad sat with his arms crossed, defiant.

"This is certainly a delicious breakfast," Bill encouraged.

"Eat it, Brad," I urged firmly.

"I'm *not* going to." Tears came to his eyes. We tried coaxing. He repeated, "I'm *not* going to eat it."

"Aw, c'mon, Brad," Zac pleaded, "Mother worked hard to cook us a nice breakfast."

Brad sobbed and shook his head vigorously.

Bill gently touched his hand. "Son, who's on the throne of your life this morning?"

Brad, pouting, replied, "The 'debil' and me."

In a quiet voice, Bill asked, "Who do you *want* on the throne?"

Brad sobbed, "Jesus."

"Then let's pray."

We sat in silence and waited. Brad's tiny voice finally trembled, "Dear Jesus, forgive me for being bad and help me to like this old egg." He picked up his fork and started to eat. He didn't stop until he had downed every bite.

That night when we had our devotions together, Bill asked, "Who was on the throne of your life today?"

"Jesus!" Zac answered.

"Jesus!" Brad echoed with a smile. "'cept for breakfast."

We may not wish to admit it, but the desire for dominance plays a large role in all of our lives. Often conflicts between spouses reflect this struggle. But when

Christ truly controls our lives and marriage, the power of the Holy Spirit enables us to resolve our differences and live in harmony.

That's why we believe the Throne Check is absolutely necessary to a happy marriage. We encourage you to apply it regularly. You will discover, as we have, that growing together spiritually will give you the deepest intimacy you can experience. And it will provide the foundation for agreement on the basic principles of stewardship so vital to preventing or reducing many of the stresses in marriage.

## For Reflection, Discussion and Action

1. It has been said that rigid rules cannot dictate how couples grow in God's Word. How are you and your spouse growing in God's Word?

2. Have you used the Throne Check to prevent potential problems in your marriage? If this concept is new to you, how will you utilize it? (Give a specific problem area in your marriage as an example.)

3. Review the five biblical truths that will help you build a Spirit-filled marriage. Together with your spouse, determine a plan of action that will help you grow in these areas.

# 9

# *Agree on Stewardship Principles*

"Give the money to Campus Crusade?" Vonette questioned, tears in her eyes. "It was a personal gift to you, Bill. From a friend whom you led to the Lord! God gave us the money for our vacation."

"But honey," I countered gently. "This is $250." I reminded her of Campus Crusade's policy at that time of accepting no more than $50 per year in personal gifts. Together with our leadership we had taken this course of action to encourage staff members to live a simple lifestyle and avoid the temptation to add to our monthly support by encouraging friends to give "extras." I asked, "Are we going to violate that policy?"

Vonette remained firm. Money had been tight, especially with the expense of raising two growing boys. Both of us had been working hard and needed a rest. For several weeks, I had sensed that the Lord wanted me to write a book about how to live the Spirit-filled life, and I needed time away from our hectic schedule to complete it.

Another friend had invited us to use his beach home

in Southern California. So we took a few days off for rest
combined with work. I spent most of my waking hours writing that book, but even so, we relaxed, had few interruptions and enjoyed being away from the office and our daily
responsibilities.

When we returned home, I kept thinking about the
$250 gift. It would have helped defray the costs of our trip.
But since we as staff had made a commitment not to accept
anything over $50 as gifts for an entire year, I felt we could
not accept the money without violating policy and displeas-
ing the Lord. Further, if I violated our policy, I could not
expect the rest of our staff to respect it.

Vonette didn't see it this way. "Didn't God miraculously provide the funds when we needed them? Would you
have been able to finish the book without the time off?
Didn't both of us need that vacation? Didn't we return
relaxed and spiritually stronger?"

But I still felt strongly that we should give the money
to the ministry.

Three days later, while we were at our staff conference, Bill asked me for the checkbook. From the set of
his jaw and his tone of voice, I knew what he intended to
do. I tried again to convince him I was right. This time, I
had an additional argument. "If you write out a check for
that amount, it will lower our bank balance almost to zero."

But Bill still insisted. Needing to leave immediately
for our staff meeting, we didn't have time to discuss the
matter further.

When he spoke that morning, the audience of staff and
friends hung on every word. *That hypocrite!* I huffed. *These
people don't really know him like I do.* Feeling my resentment build, I slipped out of the meeting to keep from
making a statement I would regret.

When we prayed before going to bed in our room that evening, I again told Bill he was wrong to return the check.

His response surprised me. "Honey, I wrote it out but didn't mail it. I couldn't until we resolve our differences. Why don't we ask God to show us what to do?"

Bill prayed aloud first. I followed. But I silently added, *If Bill is right, take all thought of this money from me. I can't handle this issue on my own any longer.*

When I finished, Bill wrapped me in his arms and assured me of his love and concern. We agreed to do what God directed. I admired my husband for that. Although we disagreed, and though I thought he was a hypocrite earlier in the day, I now felt blessed to be his wife.

Late the next afternoon in a conversation with a friend with a similar problem, I suddenly realized that the amount of money didn't matter any more. God had removed it from my mind. In a marvelous way the Lord had turned my critical, judgmental spirit toward my husband into an understanding—even loving—appreciation.

Later, with my encouragement, Bill mailed the check. And you know what? We didn't suffer any financial inconvenience.

Agreeing on how to handle money may be one of the most stressful problems for a couple. In fact, conflict over finances is a frequent cause of divorce.

## Responsibilities of Stewardship

In the last chapter we highlighted two major avenues leading to the effective management of stress in marriage:

1. *Vital spiritual life*

2. *Godly stewardship*

Now we are ready to look at the second road. If our goal is to prevent unnecessary conflict or reduce the potential for friction in our relationship, we must agree on basic principles of *godly stewardship of time, talent and treasure.* *

A steward is one who oversees the affairs of a household or estate, or manages the accounts and property of another person.

A faithful steward manages his time, talent and treasure for maximum effectiveness in doing God's will. One can determine much about a couple's spiritual life by what they treasure.

Their use of time, talents and money clearly shows their spiritual commitment because where their heart is, their treasure will follow.[1]

God is the source and owner of all we possess. All that we have, we own under God. He has put into our hands the administration of all He owns. Over the years, Bill and I have found that putting God first in our time, talents and treasure must be the goal of our stewardship. Once this is so, all else falls into place.

Our Lord addressed the importance of stewardship when He said, "Blessed is that servant whom his master will find so doing when he comes."[2] As we obey His command to faithful stewardship, we too will receive the commendation of the Master.

## Good Stewardship Is Not Easy

Living on the fast track, couples often find it difficult to follow good stewardship principles in their marriage. Many stressors detract them from the godly management of their resources. Bill examines three of those:

---

* For a complete discussion on these principles, I encourage you to read my book, *As You Sow: the Adventure of Giving by Faith* (Here's Life Publishers).

## 1. Managing Time

Early in my Christian experience, I learned that the secret to preventing stress in the use of time is to cast all our cares on the Lord.

For example, one morning I had an appointment for an interview at 8 o'clock. I received several crucial overseas calls that delayed me. Instead of fretting, I remembered, *The God who guides the universe and holds it together by His command is in control of my time, too. He's allowed these interruptions. My worrying won't change anything—except delay me longer.*

I had no alternative but to arrive late for my appointment. I explained my tardiness to the interviewer, and he graciously accepted my apology.

I don't like to keep people waiting, but I've learned to relax when I can't do anything to change the situation. If I attempt to honor my commitments, my faith helps assure me that God will work everything out. After all, that's the promise of Romans 8:28.

Busyness—a lifestyle of running from place to place, hurrying to the next project, glancing at a wristwatch every few minutes—can devastate a marriage. Your intimacy needs unhurried growth. Develop a schedule that places priority on your relationship. Manage your time to give your marriage adequate attention. God doesn't want your life so packed with activity that you lack sufficient togetherness with the one you love.

## 2. Managing Talents

God has given each of us at least one special ability. We would be poor stewards if we ignored that talent. God expects us to develop our gift to its fullest potential through the control and empowering of the Holy Spirit. Failing to do so leaves us feeling frustrated and unfulfilled.

Sometimes, however, stress comes when we over-commit ourselves in using our talents. A husband's expertise, for example, may lie in financial management—but he'll spend too many hours helping the church with its annual budget. A wife's gift in music may keep her on the road most weekends putting on concerts.

A faithful steward maximizes his abilities for God's glory. God is pleased when we encourage each other to use our talents. But He doesn't expect us to neglect our greatest gift—each other—in the process.

### 3. Managing Finances

Much sorrow in marriage stems from a lack of understanding and a failure to apply the principles of financial stewardship.

Vonette and I discovered early in our marriage that resolving financial differences begins with spiritual commitment. On that Sunday afternoon in the spring of 1951 when we decided to write our contract with the Lord, we went into separate rooms and got down on our knees to spend time alone with our Lord in prayer. We each determined to follow the example of Jesus who said that He always did what pleased the Father, and the example of the apostle Paul who referred to himself as a "slave" of Jesus Christ.[3]

Although as a businessman I had signed hundreds of agreements, I realized that this was to be the most important contract of our lives. Individually and as a couple we were surrendering ourselves totally to the Lord Jesus Christ to become His "slaves" forever.

In the contract, we vowed not to *seek* personal wealth, success, praise, honor or power for ourselves. Our document, which each of us signed, went something like this:

From this day, Lord, we surrender and relinquish

all our past, present and future rights and material possessions to You. As an act of the will, by faith, we choose to become Your bondslaves and do whatever You want us to do, go wherever You want us to go, say whatever You want us to say, no matter what it costs, for the rest of our lives. We will never seek the praise or applause of men or the material wealth of the world.

We have never regretted this commitment to our Lord. As a result of our agreement, Vonette and I personally own little of this world's goods. Yet we have always abundantly enjoyed the blessings of God which He promised to all who trust and obey Him. On thousands of occasions we have experienced the faithfulness of God to meet our every need above and beyond our fondest hopes and desires.

Though we own nothing apart from some personal effects and a modest pension for the future, I cannot think of a single thing we want that we do not have—except more finances and blessings from God to pass on to others.

## Agreeing on Stewardship Principles

We would like to share several guidelines that will help you be a good steward of your resources and prevent some of the stresses which the pressures of managing time, talents and treasure can place upon your marriage.

### 1. Apply Good Stewardship Principles

The first step in godly stewardship is to accept God's ownership over your lives and all that you possess. Dedicate your time and talents, as well as your treasures, to Him without reservation.

List your marital priorities according to biblical principles. Make the items clear and specific so you can easily follow them in your daily living. Discuss the major areas in which you disagree and ask the Holy Spirit to show you how to resolve them.

## 2. See Your Spouse as Your Partner

Partnership in stewardship is essential to marital harmony. Let me give an example.

Vonette and I believe that the most capable spouse should handle the money. As long as you have set priorities and decided on how to handle your finances, delegate the responsibility to the partner with the best aptitude for bookkeeping.

If your situation changes, switch the responsibility to the other partner. When we first married, since I was in business, I took care of our personal finances while Vonette handled the household account. As my job changed and because of my frequent travel, I found less time for such matters. I asked her to be responsible for paying our bills and keeping track of our finances.

Praying together and following the leading of the Holy Spirit, we have learned, is essential for financial agreement. When we understand that God has given us our mate to balance and complement us, we will work hard at discussing and praying over the decisions we must make.

We recommend that when disagreements come, you get down on your knees and pray together. Ask God to give you His wisdom and direction. If you still can't come together on the issue, declare a moratorium for twenty-four hours. Don't discuss the situation with each other. Talk to the Lord; ask Him to give you further insight.

If you still can't resolve the problem, try the moratorium for another twenty-four hours. For a crucial issue, we suggest you pray *and* fast. Do a Throne Check and allow God to speak to you. Examine your motives. If done with honesty, this will help you identify the problem and provide creative solutions.

### 3. Follow Biblical Guidelines for Giving

God's provision is based on the law of the harvest: *What we sow we will reap.*[4] From the seed of your giving, God will harvest bountiful fruit.

Tithing—giving at least a tenth of our income or resources to God—serves as a practical guideline for giving and ensures consistent stewardship.

The apostle Paul exhorted believers, "On every Lord's Day each of you should put aside something from what you have earned during the week, and use it for this offering. The amount depends on how much the Lord has helped you earn. Don't wait until I get there and then try to collect it all at once."[5] Without a functional plan for giving, it is easy to fall prey to the emotions and circumstances that hinder you from being faithful stewards.

Have you ever conceived grand strategies for giving, only to find that the money you intended to give vanished in day-to-day spending? Covetousness, greed, and frivolous buying all tempt even the most dedicated Christian. When budgets stretch unmanageably, many Christians skimp on their tithe to cover a personal deficit.

Since everything still belongs to God, tithing teaches us to put God first. Moses said, "The purpose of tithing is to teach you always to put God first in your lives."[6] God does not honor a gift that comes from the leftovers. He requires the first and the best of our increase.[7] Putting God first releases us from the tyranny of materialism and clears the channel for God's continued abundant blessings.

### 4. Live in Financial Freedom

Our wonderful Lord wants you to be free from financial bondage. He wants you to have enough for your household and to give joyfully and generously to God's work.

God's will about money is not a mystery. Biblical principles of stewardship give us a clear revelation of His plan. By basing your decisions on these precepts, you will experience lasting financial freedom.

I urge you to study these precepts carefully and use the "sound mind" principle of Scripture recorded in 2 Timothy 1:7.

> God has not given us a spirit of fear, but of power and of love and of a sound mind.

If necessary, seek the wise counsel of godly, successful people. Ask God to give you His peace. When you make the right decisions, you will sense incredible calm even in circumstances that seem impossible.

So many couples succumb to the lure of materialism. We need to adopt a simple lifestyle, to focus our finances on our needs, not our greeds. I recognize that we do not all share the same view of a "simple lifestyle." Ask the Lord how He wants you to define it. God wants us to enjoy pleasure and convenience. It is how we use and share our possessions that counts. Use everything to God's honor and glory and you will thwart the temptation to buy unnecessary items.

The Christian life is warfare. Perhaps the apostle Paul had this in mind when he said, "No soldier in active service entangles himself in the affairs of everyday life, so that he may please the one who enlisted him as a soldier."[8] To be an effective warrior in God's army, we must keep our material resources as free of debt as possible and use them forcefully in the war against Satan. Our lifestyle should reflect the discipline of military readiness for the moment when the Lord summons us into battle.

Let me suggest a simple formula to accomplish this goal: Give at least the first 10 percent of your income to God and save a second 10 percent for a surplus. Then live on the remaining 80 percent. If this is not possible for you, decide on a percentage for your surplus that fits your budget.

Every Christian couple should consider how they can give to help win and disciple the largest possible number of people for Christ. If every child of God would do so, vast sums of money would be available to accelerate the fulfilling of the Great Commission.

I encourage you to ask God to supply the funds to invest in His work. Look for a special project or some Christian organization which you and your spouse can support monthly, if only modestly, in addition to your commitment to your local church.

When Christ is on the throne of our lives, we have no difficulty accepting our God-given stewardship over all of life. And we see our possessions as God's gift to make us successful in ministry. By following the biblical pattern of giving, we will significantly reduce the daily stress caused by last-minute, crisis-initiated decision-making.

## For Reflection, Discussion and Action

1. If you and your spouse have not done so, dedicate your time, talents, and financial resources to the Lord. You may want to make a written contract.

2. To whom have you delegated the bookkeeping responsibilities in your marriage, and why?

3. Sit down together and look over your checkbook. Are you, as a couple, following biblical guidelines for giving? If not, how will you make adjustments to correct this situation?

# *Step 3*

## Utilize Stress-Reducers

*Through praise, communication and a healthy sex life, couples develop a sense of "otherness" which enables them to reduce stress and achieve greater wholeness and intimacy in their relationship.*

# 10

# The Power
# of Praise

During Explo '85, I was in West Berlin on the day of our thirty-seventh wedding anniversary. Vonette was in London in the video control studio which coordinated the transmission of our television broadcasts around the world via eighteen satellites.

As I stood before the packed house in the Internationalen Kongresszentrum, I remembered that this was our anniversary. On impulse, I decided to give a special anniversary greeting to Vonette. My words were carried over our worldwide television network to more than 250,000 in 98 live auditoriums with millions more listening in.

"Before I bring my message today, I want to take a moment to wish my beautiful, adorable wife of thirty-seven years a happy anniversary." The crowd went wild as I told her how much I loved and appreciated her. Cameras in the control studio in London caught her reaction and broadcast it. What a spectacular joy that was for me and the entire worldwide audience to witness her surprise and amazement.

I was thrilled to hear Bill's declaration of love on worldwide television. That was quite a public demonstration of his affection for me.

Later, when he spoke in Mexico City for the final event of the tour, many people who had viewed the broadcast wept. What touched them most was when they saw Bill's love for me after all these years. Someone mentioned later that he had praised his wife and lifted the world.

Praise is an expression of our devotion to our mate. It is the channel through which we communicate our appreciation and gratitude for each other. It is the means by which we exchange honor and respect. It is one way we share our "otherness."

## Developing "Otherness"

No marriage can succeed if either spouse insists on taking center stage. Consciously looking to the welfare of our partner first enables us to open ourselves to each other. We call this focus having a sense of "otherness."

Otherness is a basic scriptural principle. The apostle Paul urges all Christians, "Love each other with brotherly affection and take delight in honoring each other."[1] In Ephesians, he describes this precept through marital love: "Husbands should love their wives as their own bodies . . . For no man ever hates his own flesh, but nourishes and cherishes it, as Christ does the church."[2]

That's quite a comparison! We go to great lengths to care for ourselves. Stores fill their shelves with items to make us look younger and feel better. The food we eat, the clothes we buy, the way we spend our time, all focus on satisfying our own needs and desires. If we were to give as much attention to our mate as we do to the care of our own bodies, our marriage would dramatically blossom with blessings.

A sense of otherness is absolutely necessary for a healthy marital relationship. But for couples living on the fast track, otherness may be hard to cultivate.

Busy, stressful lifestyles do not lend themselves to thinking of others first. Yet self-centeredness only brings more pressure to an already strained relationship. But otherness—however difficult to develop—reduces the friction that results when we remain self-serving.

In the next three chapters, Vonette and I would like to share three major stress reducers—praise, communication and sex—that will enable you to establish or strengthen your sense of otherness and achieve greater intimacy in your relationship.

We begin with praise.

## The Selfless Qualities of Praise

The ability of an eagle to soar into the heavenlies is more than a scriptural metaphor. Spiritual and physical blessings originate in "heavenly places."[3] The flight of the eagle suggests the awesome power of praise to lift us above our stresses and into the atmosphere of God's abundant blessings.

Praise is the soul and spirit of creation. It is the natural expression of love. Vonette and I are convinced that one of the reasons our marriage is so exciting and retains its freshness is because early on we learned the power of praise and began to practice it.

By lifting our gaze heavenward, praise as a lifestyle cleanses us from self-centeredness and enables us to focus on our "otherness."

Praise, first to God and then to our mate, offers other stress-reducing benefits to marriage as well. It opens channels of communication, builds unity and harmony, enhances our mate's self-esteem and gives energy to our partnership.

Let's look briefly at each of these benefits.

## 1. Praise Opens Channels of Communication

To flow freely, the channels of communication must be cleared of their obstructions. Hostility, fear, pride, doubt, suspicion all clog the stream. Praise dissolves these blockages.

We should never speak negatively about our mate in public. I'm amazed how often spouses use subtle humor to put each other down in front of others. Concentrating on the positives in our mate, on the other hand, keeps the channels of communication open. Praise encourages this.

Sometimes Vonette expresses her displeasure over something I shouldn't have done. Instead of being confrontational, I've learned to respond with a compliment. "I'm the most fortunate man in the world to have such a wonderful wife," I smile. And I tell her how much I appreciate her for putting up with whatever it is I may be doing to irritate her. This kind of response, we have found, disarms a potentially tense situation and keeps our communication open.

## 2. Praise Builds Unity and Harmony

We have found that a lifestyle of praise to God and to our spouse helps bring unity and harmony by preparing our hearts for a deeper, more intimate relationship with God and each other. Divisions between us vanish and peace is restored when we regularly express appreciation for each other.

The reason is simple.

Thanksgiving transforms our negative dispositions into positive attitudes. We cannot truly show gratitude for the ways our partner enriches our life, then criticize him for the irritations in our marriage. I truly believe that praise encourages us to cherish each other, to focus on the positives in our relationship, thus strengthening our marital bonds.

### 3. Praise Enhances Our Mate's Self-esteem

By supporting each other through praise, we create the positive and joyful attitudes that build self-esteem.

Vonette inspires me in many ways. When I am involved in urgent matters, she stands beside me. She praises me when I've handled a situation well. She tells me I can succeed when I take on a new project.

Genuine praise always lifts those around us. When Bill expresses his appreciation for me, I feel good about myself. I have more confidence and self-respect. When I praise Bill in public, I draw attention to his strengths and abilities. Others form favorable opinions about him. This, too, helps build his self-esteem.

### 4. Praise Gives Energy to Our Partnership

Praise of God energizes our relationship with our heavenly Father. It carries our faith to His throne, surrounds our prayers with splendor, gives birth to miracles, and lifts us into a supernatural plane where Satan dare not enter.

Similarly, praise of our spouse gives energy to our partnership, bolstering our courage in stressful circumstances.

During Explo '85, Bill traveled more than 40,000 miles in four-and-a-half days and spoke twenty times. I stayed in London to help coordinate the leadership strategy.

Shortly after each daily broadcast, Bill would call.

Each time I would encourage him, "You're doing a great job." Then he would fly to the next engagement on another continent.

I came home after the event expecting to find Bill exhausted. But he was cheerful and invigorated.

"I'm so thrilled over everything that has happened," he enthused. "My last message was my best. I seemed to gather strength and energy as I traveled. You don't know how much I appreciate the encouragement you gave me all along the way."

Praise is contagious. Whenever I affirm Vonette, not only do I brighten her life, but mine as well. The dynamic energy we create keeps our relationship vital. In this atmosphere we find healing for emotional hurts and opportunity for personal growth and intimacy.

Without a lifestyle of praise, a couple cannot hope to remain close. Their lack of appreciation for each other will separate them, especially during times of stress.

## Developing a Lifestyle of Praise

Developing a lifestyle of praise is no easy task. Not only will we face Satan's resistance, but our own feelings may become an obstacle.

Feelings change and will fail us during times of stress. Have you tried to be grateful when your children come down with chicken pox, or when your husband loses his job? Do you find praise easy when your taxes are due, or when your wife wrecks the car? How do you feel when your partner is grumpy or unloving?

Making praise part of our lifestyle takes an act of the will. We cannot rely on feelings; we must consciously determine to adopt a pattern of appreciation. It all boils down to this: We can either decide to be critical, or we can choose to be complimentary. Do you want to be miserable? Then make your spouse miserable. Do you want to be happy? Then make him happy. It's your choice.

You may say, "This sounds terribly simplistic. I live in a world where this is impossible to do." Let me assure you, I had to learn this myself and it took years of practice to reach a consistent pattern of praise—and I am still learning.

Here are three practical steps you can take to make praise a way of life and reduce the stress in your marriage.

### 1. Find Qualities Worthy of Praise

I encourage you to search out qualities in your mate that are worthy of praise. If you are a person basically oriented to seeing the negative qualities in your spouse, this may be difficult. But remember the young man in Chapter 8 who did not fully appreciate his wife's beauty? He had to be reminded of it before he recognized his blindness to his wife's good qualities.

Think about it. Is your husband faithful on his job? Does he take the trash out without being asked? Does your wife fix your favorite meal? Has she accomplished a significant task on her job? Does she look particularly beautiful today? Keep these characteristics fresh on your mind. Let them supplant any temptation to criticize or tear down.

### 2. Show Gratitude Regularly

How long does your partner wait between compliments? How many times have you neglected showing appreciation for a kindness he has shown to you?

Too often we take our most precious friend—the most important person in our life—for granted.

I encourage you to show gratitude to your partner

regularly. Remember, apart from the Lord Jesus Christ, your partner is the most important person in your life — more important than your children, your parents and your business associates. Most likely you will outlive your parents. Your children will leave your nest and build their own homes. But you will be together, if you obey God, the rest of your lives. So make up your mind to enjoy that relationship. Be creative in the ways you show gratitude to your partner. Look for the ways he serves you and express your thanks.

### 3. Offer a Sacrifice of Praise

Sometimes praise calls for sacrifice.

The apostle Paul admonishes, "By Him (Jesus Christ) let us continually offer the sacrifice of praise to God, that is, the fruit of our lips, giving thanks to His name."[4] This applies to our marriage relationship as well.

Many spouses affirm each other only when it's convenient or when things are going well. But praise means so much more when it is offered during difficult times — when we are in sorrow, suffering pain, experiencing loneliness; while we're in the midst of stressful and harried circumstances.

The Scriptures record that God required Israel to bring the best of their cattle or sheep to His altar for sacrifice. The offering had to cost the penitent his choice bull or lamb. The sacrificial animal could have no defects.[5]

This principle holds true in giving praise as well. Unless our offering costs us something, it is not a sacrifice. Praise that springs sacrificially from our innermost being pleases God and enriches our marriage.

## The Next Step to Intimacy

Many couples who live on the fast track wonder where their intimacy went. Eventually the normal pressure of their world is increased by the anxiety of "We don't communicate anymore. You're so wrapped up in what you're doing that I don't seem to count. I might as well not be here."

Perhaps you have felt this way at times in your marriage.

As a stress reducer, praise is but the first step in establishing and maintaining intimacy. Vonette and I have discovered another valuable secret that will help you reduce the stress in your relationship. We want to share it with you in the next chapter.

## For Reflection, Discussion and Action

1. How have you turned a stressful experience in your marriage into an opportunity for praise?

2. Praise is the natural expression of love. Find five things worthy of praise in your spouse and share them.

3. What does it mean to offer a "sacrifice of praise?" Give an instance in your marriage in which praise was a sacrifice. How did it affect your relationship?

# 11

# *Intimacy Through Communication*

Think back to the early days of your courtship for a moment. Remember how you would sit across from each other in a restaurant, gaze into each other's eyes, and talk for hours about your hopes and dreams?

If you were like most couples in love, you just didn't have enough time for all the warm conversation the two of you wanted to share. I remember how reluctant Vonette and I were to say goodnight after a date. We had so much to talk about.

All too often, after the initial excitement of marriage wears off, husbands and wives let their intimacy decline into dull routine. As a couple who have been happily married since 1948, we know you can restore that lost sparkle of intimacy and enrich your sense of otherness if you really want to. We want to share with you the principles that have helped us build intimacy through communication and thus reduce stress in our relationship.

## Building Intimacy

Many couples equate intimacy with romance and sex. Although intimacy includes a vibrant sexual relationship and continuing romance, it covers every aspect of a couple's union.

Intimacy is a process of sharing our total selves with our partner. It includes seeking to understand the inner and outer nature of our spouse. It means revealing our most private self and giving freely of our body, mind and spirit. Intimacy comes when we know our mate thoroughly, yet love him faithfully.

Shared values and experiences, vulnerability, a sense of safety, sensitivity, loyalty, communication, forgiveness and prayer form the building blocks of closeness. The foundation upon which these qualities rest, however, is our common faith in God that allows us to risk trusting each other. The knowledge that God knows us intimately yet loves us unconditionally provides the security we need for building intimacy. Without this sense, the heart remains a lonely place.

We choose to develop this closeness, but it doesn't happen overnight. Building intimacy is a lifetime commitment that requires openness and work. The adventure is worth every moment, however, because intimacy creates a joyful oneness of heart and mind.

Time together is the mortar that holds the building blocks of intimacy in place. Marital relationships tend to deepen in proportion to the amount of time we give our mate.

Vonette and I try to make time together a priority. For example, we enjoyed a relaxing Caribbean cruise, a gift from our staff. We requested a separate table for meals aboard ship. Although that is contrary to our usual lifestyle of evangelism and discipleship, we wanted the privacy to refresh our relationship after a hectic year.

Since both of us grew up in a farming community, we also love the sights and smells of a county fair. So we attend the Los Angeles County Fair whenever possible. We stroll through the livestock exhibits and commercial buildings. We stop to see the new inventions and gadgets coming out on the market, and we view the prize-winning entries in the canning and baking contests. But most of all we enjoy the opportunity to be together.

For Bill and me the fair is a time to remember the good ole days. I remind Bill of how I won first prize for an embroidered tea towel in the third grade. He tells me again about showing livestock for his 4-H Club and how he trained the national championship livestock judging team which competed at the American Royal while he was on the faculty extension department at Oklahoma State University. We eat candy and popcorn and don't mention the word *diet.*

So we can enjoy our privacy for an extended period, we occasionally drive across country to our meetings. On our last trip, we memorized Scripture together, listened to music, and took turns driving so we could read a book aloud to each other.

The cornerstone of marital intimacy is open and loving communication. Does your relationship provide a safe haven for communication on the deepest spiritual and emotional level? Do you and your spouse freely share your dreams? Your fears? Your failures? Your successes? Can you weep together as well as laugh together? Support each other in crisis or pain?

For you "macho" men who would rather spend hours watching football or going hunting for days with your buddies, this may seem a difficult challenge. Yet we cannot build intimacy without such communication.

Silence erodes communication. I remember a time when I had a fear of death. Even though Bill and I had been married for approximately ten years and had what we felt was a good level of communication, I was trapped into silence by fear. Fear is not the most respectable problem to have, but one afternoon while he was away, I felt as if a little voice inside me were saying, "You have only two years to live." Its purpose seemed clear: to give me time to put my affairs in order. I yearned to phone Bill and share what had just occurred. But I didn't want to put another burden on him.

I tried to pass off the thought as imagination and forget it. My mind told me that such a thought was stupid. Yet my experience conditioned me to believe that everything I read was condemning—the seven virgins whose lamps were not filled with oil, the parable of the talents—and I thought I was suffering from God's judgment.

I had suffered from an ache in my shoulder for some time where a benign mole had been removed several years earlier. Was it cancer?

I decided not to tell anyone. Christ Himself would be my counselor and help me bear it.

But looking in the bathroom mirror, I could see the anxiety in my eyes and the tension lines at the corner of my mouth. I tried to shake off my feelings by telling myself I would visit a doctor soon. I pictured the Bible as a closet and searched for the right verse to clothe myself. "God has not given us a spirit of fear, but of power and of love and of a sound mind"[1] seemed appropriate.

I carried the burden of impending death through the summer months and the seasons of another year. Every unexplained throb and ache seemed like it could fulfill the prophecy.

When I lost my voice and an examination showed nodes on my vocal cords, I was sure I had cancer of the throat. At times I wanted to talk to Bill and others about it, but didn't want my problem to become a subject of gossip. The isolation of my own silence became increasingly unbearable.

Finally, I *had* to take my feelings to Bill. He listened quietly as I explained. Then he took off his suit coat and hung it on the back of the chair. He started to loosen his tie, but instead put his hands on my shoulders.

"Oh, honey, that wasn't God's voice," he said tenderly. "And you're not going to die. I've had that experience many times myself. When I'm leaving for a trip, I frequently receive an impression, *Take a good last look at Vonette and your sons; you will never see your family again.*"

Bill's compassion made me cry in relief. I had been afraid he would laugh.

"It's the subtle attack of the enemy, Vonette," Bill explained. "He tries every way possible to rob us of our peace in Christ, because the joy of the Lord is our strength."

I was the one who now reached for Bill's shoulders. My tears were gone. I felt strong again, like a deep-rooted tree that had a new ring of growth.

That moment of transparency affected us permanently as a couple. I felt a new oneness with Bill. Safe. I saw how I could trust him with my most tender (even ridiculous) feelings. The sharing gave us an overwhelming sense that we were truly partners for life.

## Intimate Communication Reduces Stress

Discussing problems lovingly and openly and being able to laugh at our mistakes decreases friction in a relationship. I'll let Bill give you an example.

One day, Vonette cleaned the closet in our guest bedroom and laid some clothes on the bed. I noticed a shirt that I liked and decided to wear it that day. But it was wrinkled, and I had just a few minutes to get ready. So I decided that since I would be wearing a coat, I could save time by only ironing the collar, cuffs and down the front. I turned on the iron, pressed a few strokes, put on the shirt and a tie, and was ready to go.

That noon we invited Kundan and Iqbal Messey, a beloved staff couple from the Middle East with whom we have served the Lord for thirty years, to be our guests for lunch. We ate on the patio. The sun was quite warm so Kundan took off his coat. As host, I felt I should follow suit. When I removed mine, everyone saw my wrinkled shirt.

Immediately, I tried to explain, but Vonette was not happy.

Bill's explanation only made things worse. I felt disgraced. Not only did this couple probably think I was negligent in caring for my husband, but Bill admitted he had pressed his own clothes. Kundan and Iqbal's culture frowned on that.

I exclaimed, "Bill, you did not have to iron your shirt! You have forty ironed shirts (a slight exaggeration) in the closet. Why would you take time to press a shirt when you have all those others you could have worn?"

I could have carried a grudge over this incident, but as we talked about it later the whole thing struck us as funny. Bill Bright, the president of Campus Crusade, ironing his own clothes! We laughed.

I appreciate Bill's willingness to talk when things like this happen. We learn so much about each other when we get our irritations and worries out into the open.

## How to Build Intimacy Through Communication

Using communication effectively to build intimacy and reduce the stress in marriage takes lots of work. But the rewards are worth the effort. Bill shares six principles that will help you in this process.

### 1. Listen

Each of us has a deep need to be heard and understood. We want to share our thoughts, feelings and ideas. But communication is first listening.

When we truly listen to our partner, we give of ourselves and focus on our mate. We understand his point of view and build his self-esteem. We communicate our love and encourage intimacy.

As you and your partner talk together, take time to understand. Ask questions. Give your undivided attention and don't interrupt unless necessary.

I sometimes read a newspaper while Vonette talks. When she gets upset, I tease, "I have two eyes and two ears. I can do several things at once."

But one day she turned the tables on me. And when I couldn't get her attention, I didn't appreciate it one bit. Now I understand how much she needs my whole self when she has something to say. Ever since, we have made a joke about getting one another's undivided attention.

I especially encourage husbands to take time to listen to their wives. Men, provide your wife with a safe harbor for sharing her concerns. Resist the temptation to use this respite for romance or sex. Simply commit yourself to listening. You may find that this means going to a neutral place like a restaurant so your wife is free from normal distractions.

## 2. Speak Gently

I hate to throw anything away, even socks—especially if they're my favorite. One morning I slipped on a pair that had a weak elastic top. So I used a safety pin to hold one up.

Vonette's sharp eye noticed it. "Why are you wearing a safety pin in your sock?"

"The elastic's loose."

"Why don't you throw them away?"

"But I've had these for fifteen years."

She laughed. "Well, Bill Bright, after fifteen years they deserve to be retired! It wouldn't be worth my time to fix them. If I sewed elastic inside the sock, you wouldn't wear it."

"But they're still good socks!" I insisted. "They don't have any holes. The only problem is, they droop."

To me, pinning up a prize sock was no big deal. But to Vonette, her value as a wife was at stake. She was looking at my sock and thinking, *Oh, man, that makes me feel guilty.* To have a pin in my sock signaled to her that Bill Bright needed attention.

For many couples, such differences in values could cause stress. These little conversations could turn into angry confrontations. Words can inflict pain, unless we speak them gently. And sometimes with humor. We have smoothed many potential conflicts in our relationship with humor and by being gentle in our responses.

The Scripture is full of advice on controlling our tongue. The psalmist urges, "Keep your tongue from evil."[2] Proverbs says, "A soothing tongue is a tree of life."[3]

A soothing tongue refrains from making accusations. In discussing your differences, attack the problem, not the person. Use pleasant words with a gentle tone of voice.

Have an open, understanding mind. Try to appreciate everything you can about your partner's point of view. Interject humor to ease the strain.

## 3. Communicate Through Touch

Touching says what words cannot.

When Vonette rubs my back, I feel special and respond like a cat having his fur stroked. If we sit near each other, we move close to share our oneness.

We often hold hands when we pray to signify our unity. Vonette's warm embrace during sad experiences brings more comfort than a thousand words.

The necessity of nonsexual touching continues throughout marriage. Vonette especially likes for me to rub her neck and back vertebrae. Physical contact gives positive recognition and support and deepens intimacy in a way nothing else can.

Find unique ways of communicating with your spouse through touch. Ask your partner for positive physical contact when you need it.

## 4. Be Vulnerable

To be vulnerable we must risk revealing who we are.

This isn't easy.

We all find it hard to open ourselves to others. Sometimes we hide behind masks to avoid being hurt.

But if we put barriers between us and our partner, we will stifle communication. Our spouse will not know or understand us. He will not be able to meet our needs, or know why we react the way we do to stressful circumstances.

Keep yourself open to your partner. Accept the pain and inconvenience you may feel from your vulnerability as part of the process of building your relationship.

## 5. Forgive Freely

Genuine forgiveness is more than pretending the offense didn't happen. It is an act of the will in the power of the Holy Spirit by which we release another from his offense and surrender our hurt to God.

Forgiveness oils the conflicts in our relationship. It allows us to be vulnerable to each other and keep our intimacy growing. It helps us respond lovingly to criticism and listen to our spouse's negative remarks and learn from them. As a result, we answer calmly and quietly, not fueling the flame of ill feelings.

## 6. Pray Together

Bill and I sleep in two double beds brought together by a single headboard made by Bill's father. I sleep in one bed, he in the other. But every night before we go to sleep, we kneel to pray together on my side. Once in bed, Bill usually stays beside me until I fall asleep. Then he goes back to his bed. When we wake in the morning, we kneel to pray together again, side by side. Although our personal times with the Lord are more protracted, our times together are usually brief.

Our prayer life has increased intimacy in our communication. When we turn our burdens and conflicts over to the Lord together, we share a peace and closeness we find nowhere else in our relationship. Our prayer union gives us insight into each other's walk with the heavenly Father. We keep in touch with the most intimate spiritual part of our lives. We grow together in maturity and grace.

All the other ways we communicate are strengthened through praying together. We could not imagine intimacy without the cleansing power of talking to our Lord together.

We encourage you to develop the practice of praying

together. Invite the Holy Spirit to help you communicate clearly and lovingly. Discover the innermost secrets of your hearts together through communion with the heavenly Father.

Is intimacy through communication important in your marriage?

The joy of intimacy is inexpressible. Vonette and I are still growing closer in our relationship. And we expect to keep doing so the rest of our lives together.

We work at communicating wherever we are, verbally and nonverbally. And one of the most exciting avenues of intimate communication is through our sexual relationship. The communication we have developed through the years helps us to enjoy that area of our lives even more today than when we first married.

## For Reflection, Discussion and Action

1. Review the six principles for building intimacy. What role does communication play in your relationship?

2. Give several suggestions on how a spouse can become a good listener. How have you applied this in your marriage?

3. Give examples of how you are building intimacy with your spouse.

4. Forgiveness and gentleness lead to intimacy. Give examples of how you apply these to your marriage.

# 12

# *Sex: God's Gift for Stress Relief*

Vonette and I now are at the stage of life we used to think was too old for people to have ideas about sex. Not only do we still have ideas, we celebrate our sexuality regularly.

In fact, we are experiencing a richer, fuller sex life now than at any time in our forty-plus years together. The ways we have grown together have helped to make our physical relationship what it is today.

Sex should be the most intimate experience in the marriage relationship. All the other qualities of a successful marriage — intimacy, partnership and communication — contribute to a healthy sex life, making it the ultimate celebration, the icing on the cake.

No couple performs perfectly in the marriage bed from the beginning. We were no exception. By experience and experimentation, we learned to make our sexual life more loving, tender and fulfilling.

The secular media pictures sex as casual and need-driven. Hollywood tries to tell us that all we need to feel

ecstasy and fulfillment is a man, a woman and passion.
They want us to believe that sex is an instinct we cannot
control. But God's Word offers a totally different view—sex
is a gift from God meant exclusively for partners in marriage.

## The Spirituality of Sex

Sex was God's idea from the beginning. He created the
human body with its desires and called it good. He did not
make certain parts of our nature honorable and others evil.

If God equipped us with needs and desires, would He
then forbid us to satisfy them? Of course not. He designed
us to live together in marriage and become "one flesh."[1]

God's Word talks about sexual intercourse simply as
"to know."[2] This implies the most intimate knowledge of a
partner possible. God understood the beauty of getting to
know one person in a deeply intimate way and formed us
to express our romantic love physically.

But romantic love is more than physical. Our sexual
and spiritual lives are linked. The marriage bond between
a husband and wife symbolizes a believer's spiritual union
with our Lord Jesus Christ.

The apostle Paul drew this parallel in his Second
Epistle to the Corinthians, "I am jealous for you with a
godly jealousy; for I betrothed you to one husband, that to
Christ I might present you as a pure virgin."[3] To the
Ephesians he declared, "That the husband and wife are one
body is proved by the Scripture which says, 'A man must
leave his father and mother when he marries, so that he
can be perfectly joined to his wife, and the two shall be one.'
I know this is hard to understand, but it is an illustration
of the way we are parts of the body of Christ."[4]

The sexual side of marriage is the culmination of marital partnership. Nowhere else do we express our unity more

fully than through this union. Both partners become givers and receivers. Their relationship attains its highest meaning and beauty when they offer their partnership to God who brought them together as one.

That's why we consider sex an act of worship. If either of us use our physical affection for purely lustful desires, then it becomes ugly and selfish. But when our lovemaking expresses reverence to God and thankfulness for each other, it becomes a worshipful experience — though we concentrate on making sex playful, fun and satisfying.

We have learned that it is as important to be filled with the Spirit in bed as when preaching a sermon or teaching a Sunday school class. Because sex bonds a couple spiritually as well as physically, they share more than a moment of pleasure; they experience a wholeness in their relationship that only the Spirit of God can create. Sex outside of marriage violates the law of God, grieves the Holy Spirit and robs the participants of this blessedness.

Vonette and I share a joyful celebration of love. Often I have told her, "Sometimes I have to pinch myself; is it really true that we have enjoyed sex only with each other more than forty years?" We savor our physical affections more today than when we were first married.

This all sounds so wonderful and easy. Yet during periods of high stress, many couples decrease the frequency of making love. But marriage partners can enjoy God's delightful gift to reduce the stress.

## Stress-Reducing Qualities of Sex

Sex is one way husbands and wives can come together completely and shut out the rest of the world. People ask us, "How do you maintain a healthy relationship with so little time together?" "How can you handle the stress of living in a fish bowl?" We answer, "Because there are times when we go into our bedroom and shut the door. We're totally alone. We play and have fun."

Have you ever thought, *Our sex life is so routine, I can predict every second of our time together?* Or, *Our sex life lost its magic years ago?*

Like anything else in marriage, physical affection takes time and thought. We want to suggest some practical ways in which a healthy sexual relationship can reduce stress and build your intimacy as a couple.

## 1. Keep Romance Alive

Sexual love is both romance and physical satisfaction. They cannot be separated without leaving a void. And usually the little things that bring a tender aura are the first to be crowded out of a busy couple's life.

How can one heighten romance in marriage? Vonette shares valuable insights on this.

First, *make the bedroom the most beautiful room in the house.* Decorate it with feminine touches and loveliness.

Don't use the bedroom as a study or workroom. That only makes it more difficult to shut out your stresses and fill the room with romance. Instead, reserve this special place as a fun and secure haven for the two of you.

Second, *wives, wear feminine nightclothes.* Negligees should be among the most lovely and special pieces in your wardrobe. Save your favorite gown for romantic evenings to heighten your sense of awareness every time you put it on.

Third, *take every precaution for good daily hygiene.* Nothing cools a romantic feeling more than bad breath or uncleanliness. Use your regimen to entice your partner.

Fourth, *create a romantic atmosphere.* Bill and I have

found that romantic music and flowers and other thoughtful touches really do make a difference.

Romance in marriage is an individual preference.
Study your mate to discover the little things that turn his
sexual experience into the most pleasure. Prepare ahead of
time for those special touches that make him tingle and feel
loved.

## 2. Overcome Obstacles to Sexual Intimacy

For the couple on the fast track, many obstacles stand
in the way of a satisfying romantic sexual interlude. Let me
suggest several ways you can handle these barriers.

First, *deal with your fatigue.* Exhaustion can be a
major obstacle to sexual love. Manage your activities so that
you have enough vigor for physical love. Put off a few chores
until the next day. Hire a babysitter to give you time alone.
Relax and rest together. Make love in the morning when
you feel more refreshed.

Second, *guard your privacy.* If you constantly battle
interruptions during your intimate moments, romance will
fade. Sometimes simple preparations will ensure your
privacy.

Put a lock on the bedroom door. Fearing the intrusion
of a child during lovemaking can inhibit freedom of expression.

Take the telephone off the hook.

Spend an evening away together.

Use your imagination to carve out places and times in
which you can be alone.

Third, *be creative.* Routine takes its toll on all of us.
Avoid sameness in your lovemaking. Imagine new ways to
give your partner pleasure. Read a book together on sexual
techniques to bring spice into your relationship. Consider
your lovemaking an adventure and set out to discover all

you can about your partner's desires.

Fourth, *deal with negative feelings before you enter the bedroom.* Depression, anger, resentment or selfishness will thwart your sexual intimacy. Build time into your evening to talk over your problems. Use the Throne Check. Keep channels of communication open during your time together by practicing forgiveness and by supporting and nurturing your partner.

### 3. Balance Sexual Desire With Companionship

A fulfilling sexual relationship, we have said, doesn't begin in bed. True lovemaking is the culmination of an entire day (or longer) of companionship. Bill shares helpful insights on this.

First, *keep in touch when you are apart.* Whenever possible locally, call your mate at least once or twice a day just to say, "I love you." Wives, don't wait for him to take the initiative. When he travels, anticipate your reunion. Plan for his return by fixing his favorite meal or buying a small gift. Husbands, when you're away, send romantic cards and shop for special gifts that express your love but are not necessarily expensive.

Second, *don't violate your partner's trust.* Trust and intimacy are closely linked. When we build emotional stability, we provide a safe place for intimacy to grow.

Vonette and I have a rule when we travel: Neither of us spends time alone with someone of the opposite sex. No matter where we are, we don't show undue affection for anyone else. And, if necessary, we gently rebuff any unseemly actions from others.

We have committed ourselves to remain faithful to each other until death. I tell Vonette, "I'd rather die than be unfaithful to you." And she knows I mean it.

On countless occasions I have prayed, "Father, if there is a chance that I will bring dishonor to You by being unfaithful to Vonette, please take my life first." God has graciously kept us faithful to Him and to each other since that wonderful day when we said, "I do, until death do us part." We both know, however, how weak and vulnerable our fleshly natures can be. That's the reason it's so important to live in the fullness and control of the Holy Spirit. Only God can enable us to be faithful. We trust Him to continue to keep us true to Him and each other.

Third, *show respect for your partner.* Many relationships are damaged by one partner's disregard for the other's feelings. A husband may make negative remarks about his wife in public. A wife may ridicule her husband's characteristics to a friend.

Belittling each other inhibits sexual intimacy. On the other hand, showing respect—in public or private—creates trust and builds confidence.

Be sensitive to the moods and feelings of your mate. When your husband comes home after a pressure-filled day, give him the attention he needs. When your wife has had a devastating day, build her up. Put your spouse at ease by the tender things you do and say. Let him know that being with him is the best part of your day. Make your partner your best friend, in the bedroom and out.


Fourth, *keep humor in your relationship.* Humor reduces stress and heightens the fun a couple can enjoy together. Bill has a way of disarming me with his sense of humor. One day I pointed out—maybe a little too harshly—"You spilled gravy on your tie."

A sly look crept across his face. "I don't think a wife should be critical with a husband when he gets food on his tie," he responded. "All he has to do is put the tie in the refrigerator to keep the food from spoiling."

How could I stay irritated? I had to laugh.

Fifth, *do special things for each other.* There are many little things we can do for our partner. If his shirts need buttons, sew them on. Take the time to prepare a candlelight dinner. Fix breakfast and bring it to your spouse in bed. Use timely bits of praise and communication to deepen your intimacy.

Surprise adds an element of newness and innovation to a relationship. Bring home flowers. Buy her favorite perfume. The list of surprises is endless. Unexpected pleasures and deeds will heighten your anticipation of sex immensely.

Sixth, *play together.* A dear friend led a very disciplined life. He read his Bible daily, jogged regularly, and worked hard. But his schedule left no room for his wife's needs. Finally, his marriage virtually crumbled.

Realizing his error, he rearranged his schedule. He studied his Bible at a more convenient time. He cut down on the many hours he was exercising. Although he continued to work hard, he began to spend time at home doing fun things with his wife.

Their nonsexual play soon increased their desire for each other, and their sexual life began to improve dramatically.


Vonette and I have discovered that our sexual relationship demands our deepest commitment to each other. But the benefits we receive—a secure partnership, firmly established priorities and a thriving intimacy—bring high satisfaction and enable us to reduce the stresses we experience.

In the preceding chapters we have presented three of

the five steps for recognizing and managing the stresses in marriage—*enter into a partnership, establish God-centered priorities,* and *utilize stress reducers.* Another pressure on couples is how to handle the tensions of family while living on the fast track. In the coming pages we will discuss principles to help you manage the stresses of parenting, enable you to cope with inevitable family crises, and bring balance to your busy life.

## For Reflection, Discussion and Action

1. Review the concepts on the spirituality of sex. How can these affect your marriage relationship in a positive way?

2. What creative ideas can you employ to keep the romance in your relationship despite your busy schedule?

3. Trust and intimacy are closely linked. What elements in your marriage are preventing the growth of trust and intimacy?

# *Step 4*

## Handle the Stress of Family

*When couples accept their children as God's plan for their child-rearing years, they can hang tough through family crises and keep their relationship vibrant during extended periods of stress.*

# 13

# *The Stress of Children*

Just as we were ready to leave, a famous coach who had traveled across the country to California for the Rose Bowl arrived at Arrowhead Springs unannounced. He had driven a long way just to chat with me.

I faced a real dilemma. I wanted to visit with this great coach, whom I truly admired, but I also wanted to get away with my sons. Should I tell him that I didn't have time and risk offending him? Or should I put the boys off until another day?

## Rearing Children in a Busy Household

Parenting poses special problems for busy couples. The tension between ministry or business demands and the children's need for loving attention frequently places burdens on the family. Working couples often must juggle responsibilities or decide issues not faced by traditional families. They have less time and energy to spend in rearing children. A colicky baby, a hyperactive child, or a troublesome teenager can significantly increase the pressure on them. Soon their partnership suffers and the family feels the consequences.

Did you feel about parenting as I did before the arrival of our first child? Did you have idealistic lists of "do's and don'ts" to turn out well-adjusted, mature young adults? How terrifying it must have seemed when few of those "do's and don'ts" applied.

Many prospective parents fail to realize that parenting is at least a twenty-year task involving intensive work and attention. Expecting to easily adjust to the little one joining their twosome, they don't prepare adequately for extensive changes. Soon they are knee-deep in diapers, bottles and babysitters' telephone numbers. They can't see an end in sight, and wonder how they could have stumbled into such a pressure-filled lifestyle.

Busy couples face a myriad of stressors which threaten their partnership and create tensions within the family. Physical distress, emotional strain, financial pressure, religious conflict and loss of intimacy are among the major stressors.

## Coping With the Stress of Parenting

Parenting is a complex art, but you can ease the pressure if you practice the skills designed to help you handle stressful family situations. Vonette and I have found the challenges of parenting not only surmountable but have used them to enrich our family life. She shares six practical guidelines that will enable you to significantly reduce the stress:

### 1. Realize that Children Are a Gift of God

In today's pull-apart world, many parents regard their children as nuisances. But God's Word says, "Children are a gift of God; they are his reward."[1] Although children often cause stressful moments in our lives, seeing them as God's gifts and not nuisances to push aside gives us a godly and positive perspective on parenting.

## 2. Give Your Partner Top Priority

Nothing builds this security for children more than a loving relationship between their parents. Your child's most fundamental sense of love and security will come from watching how you and your spouse relate to one another. A nurturing marital partnership provides fertile soil for your child to grow and achieve independence. So let him have no doubt that your spouse is the number one person in your life, aside from the Lord Jesus.

## 3. Trust God for Your Children

Entrusting God with your children will help defuse the anxiety you feel over their future and enable you to react in difficult situations with a godly perspective.

Children have a free will. At one point in their lives they must decide whether to receive Jesus Christ as their Savior and Lord. They must choose either to live a carnal or a fruitful, Spirit-filled life. Young people from godly homes sometimes go astray despite their parents' best efforts to rear them in the nurture and admonition of the Lord. Most often, however, this is not the case.

When Zac and Brad were small, Bill and I often heard stories about how children of other Christian leaders didn't follow the Lord. Some families seemed to encounter one problem after another because the parents were so involved in Christian work. Consequently, we were concerned about failing our children in some way. We discussed this issue many times.

Then one day, I asked a respected pastor's advice. "Do you think I am making a mistake by being so involved in Bill's ministry?"

He wisely answered, "Vonette, those children belong to God and will turn out the way He directs. As long as you do what He wants, you can trust Him with your sons."

Then I began to notice how many lay people have similar problems. I realized that a parent's station in life matters less than his commitment to his children and to the heavenly Father.

We're not saying that your actions will not influence your children. The opposite is true. But when you commit yourself to the Lord and your partner and obey scriptural commands in parenting, you can be at peace that whatever happens in your family is part of God's plan.

## 4. Give Your Children Adequate Attention

This means investing time on a daily basis to encourage them, instruct them, listen to them, and share special moments with them.

Involve your children in all major family decisions including moving, larger purchases likes houses and cars, planning family outings and vacations. And when you set aside a time for fun together, don't disappoint them. Give them top priority for that occasion.

Bill could easily have postponed his mountain trip with Brad and Zac to meet with the football coach. Instead, he visited with the coach for a few minutes, then tactfully explained—in the presence of our children—his prior commitment and set off to enjoy a day of nature with his two favorite guys. And what a time they had!

How long has it been since you put down the newspaper or turned off the TV and sat down face to face to share with your children? Have you praised them recently for good behavior or complimented them for a task well done? Can they count on you to be there for them when they have a problem?

Just being "on deck" for your children means a lot. When our boys were young, for example, Bill would come home for dinner even though his work wasn't finished. He would often wrestle with them or engage in fun games until they went to bed, then go back to the office and complete his work. Not only did He feel refreshed after having such a wonderful break, he also shared the best part of our sons' day. He got to enjoy a meal with us and then tuck them into bed.

Even when he was traveling the world, Bill was always available to the boys and me. I knew he would catch the next plane home if we needed him.

## 5. Use Godly Principles in Disciplining Children

Like every other family, we had problems with discipline. We did not raise two boys who reached sainthood before the age of five. When they were young, Bill often found it necessary to spank them or correct them in other ways. But we tried to follow three rules in the process:

First, *we tried never to discipline the boys when we were angry.* The purpose of discipline is not to vent wrath, but to correct and instruct. Anger provokes children and teaches them to fear. We asked the Lord to help us correct our children in a biblical way.

When Brad misbehaved, for example, either Bill or I would talk with him.

"Brad, you know you've been disobedient."

"Yes . . . "

"You deliberately ignored our directions, didn't you?"

This time perhaps only a nod.

"When you break a rule, what happens?"

"You have to spank me."

"Why do I discipline you?"

"Because you love me."

The conversation didn't always go that smoothly, but early on we had explained to our sons that God disciplines us when we are disobedient because He loves us.[2] We tried to reinforce this with the boys until they understood why they had to be corrected.

Second, *we apologized for mistakes.* When Zac was a junior in high school, he had an appointment with his orthodontist. Before he left, I reminded him, "Don't forget your retainer. The dentist has to check it."

That afternoon I picked him up at school to take him to the doctor. On the way, I asked, "You brought your retainer, didn't you?"

"Oh, Mother, I forgot," he groaned.

"Where is it?"

"At home."

I felt irritated. "I reminded you to take it this morning. Now we don't have time to run home to pick it up." My anger mounted. "You could have called me. But no, you didn't even *think* about the trouble you've caused."

Suddenly, it seemed as if God pointed a finger at me. "You are certainly not modeling a good example as a mother." Mentally I replayed the words I had spoken to Zac.

"I'm sorry," I sighed to him. "I've been hard on you. I shouldn't have gotten angry. When I tried to help you learn to be more responsible, I lost my temper."

Zac smiled. "That's okay." A few minutes later he said softly, "I'm sorry about forgetting. I'll try to do better next time."

My apology brought out the best in Zac and helped him to see that parents can admit when they are wrong. When I stopped the car at the orthodontist's office, he ran to the other side to help me out. He opened the door to the office and made sure I had a place to sit. He even picked out a magazine for me to read.

Third, *we tried to follow through once we set rules.* Bill and I discovered this wasn't easy to do.

For example, when Zac was two years old, he began to assert his independence. He deliberately spilled his milk on the floor. I spanked him. In anger, he threw a package of napkins into the milk.

"Zac, pick them up," I said firmly.

He didn't budge.

"If you don't, I'll have to spank you again."

He shook his head. I picked up a small paddle and used it once. He still refused to obey. Another swat, followed by continued stubbornness.

Bill and I were in a difficult position. Our son was determined to assert his will. We could have given in, picked up the napkins and soothed, "Okay, but next time . . . "

It was quite a scene. Zac was sobbing, then Bill and I were crying. This went on for several minutes. Finally, I took his hand and made him bend down to pick up the napkins.

Then we both hugged him. We tried to explain why we insisted that he obey. At two years of age he probably didn't understand all we told him. But we weren't disciplining for the moment; we were looking to the years ahead and adulthood.

Parental authority, however, should never be used to control your own stress. Always try to evaluate your discipline for the good of your children, not your own convenience. Help them understand clearly what you expect of them. And make sure your rules and standards provide a proper atmosphere for their development.

## 6. Provide a Stable Home Environment

As Christian parents, we have a serious responsibility to provide a stable home environment.

One of the best ways to accomplish this is to model Christ-like love. Since children are prone to emulate our perceptions, prejudices and preferences, we need to look at the way we treat them, examine our actions toward them and others, and check our attitude toward the world.

Setting limits adds stability to a home environment as well. A survey among the most well-adjusted children in a school found three things all the children had in common: (1) their parents loved each other; (2) the children knew they were wanted and loved; and (3) discipline was consistent. According to the survey, children who know their boundaries feel secure about their place in life.

As your children grow older, expand their boundaries to give room for growth and maturity. Explain why you curtail certain activities, especially during adolescence. This helps them see that the rules are for their benefit, not yours.

## Parenting Comes Once in a Lifetime

Vonette and I have discovered that parenting is a seasonal responsibility. For most of us it comes once in a lifetime. But the payoffs are tremendous.

One day after he had married Terry, Zac phoned me. "Dad, I want two days of your time."

"That's wonderful! What did you have in mind?"

"The first day," he explained, "I want you to share the most important things you've learned in your Christian life. The second day, I want you take me witnessing and teach me more about how to talk to others about Jesus Christ."

Can you imagine how honored I felt? Zac's desire to spend two days sharing my life spoke volumes about his regard for me. Nothing could have made me more proud as a father.

Those two days made our relationship closer than ever before. I shared everything I could about my life with Jesus—the lessons I had learned, the principles I live by, and why they were important to me. We had a wonderful day of witnessing together, sharing Christ with several who had not yet received Him as their Savior and Lord. What father could ask for more than that?

Our children have been a great blessing to us. Brad and Zac taught us much about sharing, loving, patience, listening and understanding. And how to adjust and become flexible.

Vonette and I would hate to think of the kind of people we might be today without the lessons we learned as parents. Our experience reminded us often of our shortcomings and made us more dependent on the Lord for His help.

By following the guidelines we have discussed, you too can manage the stress of children and keep your marriage vibrant. Through difficulties and pressure, you can build eternal values into your children that will continue long after you are gone. These will be passed on to your children's children for generations.

## For Reflection, Discussion and Action

1. In what area is your family experiencing stress today? How will you deal with the stress?

2. Think about your relationship with your spouse.

Are you giving your partner top priority as you deal with the stress of parenting? If not, what steps can you take toward this goal?

3. For busy couples, consistency in training and discipline of children is hard to perform. How can biblical principles for raising children help you to be more consistent?

# 14

# *Managing Family Crises*

Nothing makes a couple feel more helpless than the illness of a child.

I remember when Zac, at three weeks of age, was unable to digest his formula. Bill and I took him to the doctor.

His first diagnosis was that the milk disagreed with his system. So we tried goat's milk and several other formulas which the doctor prescribed as more digestible.

During the next couple of weeks, Zac's condition grew much worse and we were frightened over his condition. The doctor was also alarmed.

"Your baby has an obstruction of his digestive system called pyloric stenosis," he announced. "You must take him to Children's Hospital immediately. We have to operate before he gets dehydrated."

In those days, many medical experts didn't think it wise for parents to stay with their sick child, nor were there any provisions for parents to remain overnight with their children. "There's no need for you here," the nurse at the hospital informed us as she took our baby from our arms. "The best thing you can do is go home and make yourself busy. We'll call you when your child is out of surgery."

After saying goodbye to our tiny son, we walked down the sidewalk together, crying. Neither of us knew if we would ever see him alive again. "Lord, we need Your help," we pleaded. "Please heal our dear little lad."

When we were able to visit Zac after the surgery, his hands and feet were tied down to keep his body straight so the incision could heal properly. He had cried so much that he could only make gasping sounds. We ached to reach down and cradle him.

How hard it was to watch him struggle in that lonely room for a long week. It wrenched our hearts to have to leave him at night. We continually had to draw upon the Lord's power for strength.

Into each of our lives come unavoidable and unexpected adversities that disrupt our lives, strain our relationships and leave us with haunting memories. Some crises last a few hours; others go on for years. Yet each gives us the breathless sense of being out of control.

How do we respond to traumatic events? Must we sit quietly and watch stressful circumstances tear our family apart? Or do we use them to enrich our marriage?

## Hanging Tough Through Crises

Crises come in many forms and affect families differently from the normal stresses of everyday life. Knowing how to cope can mean the difference between letting a catastrophe cripple our family and growing through our difficulties. Bill shares three principles that will help you manage the devastating events in your life and keep your marriage vibrant during rough times:

## 1. Maintain a Vital Spiritual Relationship

Difficult times of heartache and sorrow are the usual experience for everyone, including those who love the Lord.

Job, for example, lost his wealth and children. King David felt deep sorrow over the death of his infant son. Ruth chose to leave her people and country to follow her beloved mother-in-law.

The apostle James exclaims, "Consider it all joy, my brothers, whenever you face trials of many kinds, because you know that the testing of your faith develops perseverance. Perseverance must finish its work so that you may be mature and complete, not lacking in anything."[1]

Our obedient walk with God is not a guarantee that we will never experience painful circumstances. Instead, our Lord often uses difficult times to prune and shape us to be more like Jesus Christ. But He promises to be with us, assuring us of His peace and joy.[2]

Read through the list of persevering saints mentioned in Hebrews 11:32-39. God did not deliver them—even from death—but He commends them for their faithfulness.

Do you view crisis as a time of danger and heartache? Or do you see it as an opportunity to expand your faith and become all that God has planned for you to be? Crisis stimulates spiritual growth.

In facing adversity, we need an eternal perspective. It's easy to get so bogged down in the swirl of a crisis that we lose our spiritual moorings. We fail to manage our situation because we don't see it from God's viewpoint. Yet when we surrender our hardships to our loving, gracious and compassionate heavenly Father, our fears and disappointments shrink.

It was during "KC 83" that I experienced one of my greatest personal losses. In 1983 Campus Crusade held a student Christmas conference in Kansas City. Vonette and

I gathered with almost 20,000 staff and college students for an exciting week of training in discipleship and evangelism.

President Reagan had graciously made a videotape addressing the students. I planned to share the tape and highlights from the conference with my darling, saintly mother in Coweta, Oklahoma, only a short distance away, as soon as the conference ended. I knew she would love it.

Before the meetings began, I held a press conference. As I made my final remarks, someone handed me a note. My sister in Oklahoma was on the telephone.

Her voice quivered. "Bill, Mother just passed away. As we were talking by telephone, she told me that she was tired and wanted to take a nap before lunch. Apparently she went to sleep and while asleep went to be with the Lord."

Only a few minutes had passed after the conversation because a nurse found Mother when she brought her lunch.

I felt devastated. Although my mother was 93 years old and was eager to see her precious Savior, I would miss her terribly. I would have seen her in just a few days, but now she was gone.

Immediately, I went to my hotel room to pray. I was scheduled to give the keynote address to this great gathering of enthusiastic students that evening. But how could I? Where would I find the strength, courage and calmness I needed?

While on my knees, the Lord infused me with His strength and impressed me to give the message. I had wanted Mother to be at the conference, but she couldn't come because of her physical condition. Kneeling before the Lord, I somehow felt she wouldn't miss the meetings after all. Now she would be seeing them from her heavenly view!

So I gave my address that night. I chose to go on in the strength and peace that the Lord provided in spite of my grief.

In all our crises we must give God time to work out His purposes. As humans, we want to patch things up in a hurry and get out of our stressful circumstances.

If you are in the midst of a personal crisis, Vonette and I urge you not to make hasty decisions or consider your situation hopeless. Instead, put your trust in your loving heavenly Father to bring good out of the situation. He is full of compassion and mercy and will not abandon you.

The psalmist said, "Be delighted with the Lord. Then he will give you all your heart's desires. Commit everything you do to the Lord. Trust him to help you do it and he will."[3] As with Job, God will bring order out of chaos and turn tragedy into triumph when you remain faithful to Him, trusting, praising and thanking Him during your suffering.

## 2. Pull Together

The entire family suffers when just one member goes through a crisis. Pulling together as marriage partners is absolutely essential if we are to keep our family from splintering while under pressure. In moments of stress we must make the difficulty a dilemma to conquer together.

You will recall from Chapter 1 Vonette's telephone call to me in Brazil. I was on a month-long tour of South America, helping to launch the Here's Life World campaigns in each country. Vonette had learned that she had a tumor. Her doctor wanted to operate right away since the mass seemed to be growing rapidly. When Vonette called to tell me, I insisted on returning home immediately to be with her despite my pressing responsibilities in Brazil and other Latin countries.

"No, Bill," she insisted. "I know how crucial the Here's Life World campaign is. Millions of souls are at stake. Let me see what I can work out here."

We prayed together over long distance lines. I asked

the Lord to spare her life and keep the tumor from endangering her health.

Vonette went to another doctor for a second opinion. He confirmed the first diagnosis. After discussing her situation, the doctor agreed that Vonette could safely delay the operation to spend a few days with her parents in Oklahoma and then meet me when I arrived later in Boston where we were to speak at one of our Executive Seminars. We had a wonderful time ministering together, and I was able to share the miracles of my trip and comfort and encourage her for the coming surgery.

The day after we returned to Arrowhead Springs, Vonette entered the hospital. Our sons, Zac and Brad, joined us for fellowship and prayer. We received strength from each other. As a nurse wheeled her on a gurney toward the operating room, I walked beside her, holding her hand. Neither of us knew whether the tumor was malignant. She pressed my hand and I squeezed hers. Just before she went into the operating room, we said a final prayer together.

I went to the prayer chapel where I waited and prayed. An hour passed, then two. No word from the operating room. Two more hours went by—more than twice the time the doctors had estimated. Yet the Lord filled my heart with the assurance that He was in control.

Then the good news came! Vonette was going to be all right. The tumor was benign.

We must not underestimate the value of family support during times of crisis. Each person has a unique contribution to keep the family unit healthy and caring during hard times. Wives most often shine at preserving unity, at building esteem, at encouraging optimism and cooperation between family members. Many times husbands are best at controlling aggressive behavior and helping maintain rules and procedures that enable the family to function. Even the youngest child can add laughter and sparkle to a saddened household.

### 3. Get Help

Sometimes a crisis is so devastating, a family doesn't know how to rebuild. In this situation, spouses need to reach outside the family circle for counsel and support.

Be open about your problems and heartaches with your Christian friends. Shared spiritual commitment can bolster sagging spirits and help mend torn emotions.

Your church or community may provide programs and services for families under stress. I encourage you to find a support group that deals with crises similar to yours.

If necessary, seek professional Christian counsel. I am convinced that most of our problems can be resolved by saturating our minds with the Word of God, claiming His promises, and drawing from the supernatural resources of the risen Christ through the Holy Spirit. But sometimes only Spirit-directed Christian psychologists or pastors trained in biblical counseling can unravel the tangle of emotions wrapped around a family in crisis.

Vonette and I have seen the fruits of standing firm when life's storms rocked our frail family boat. We have watched our gracious Lord calm the winds in some situations and stand beside us to ride out the waves in others. Always, He has been faithful.

## Taking the Final Step

In this book, we have viewed four vital steps for recognizing and managing stress that will help you achieve greater intimacy in your marriage:

*Enter Into a Partnership*
*Establish God-centered Priorities*

*Utilize Stress Reducers*

*Handle the Stress of Family*

We are now ready to take the final step: *Prepare for the Golden Years.*

All of us pass through various stages in our life. Vonette and I are now experiencing one of these transitions—the golden years. Adapting to the changes which these phases create is vital to how well we manage the stresses in our marriage. In the coming pages, we want to share with you some of the lessons we are learning. We want to help you prepare for your golden years, and give you several guidelines for enjoying your marriage during this period of your life.

## For Reflection, Discussion and Action

1. How can busy couples "hang tough" through a family crisis? Give an example of how you have applied this to your relationship.

2. Think of a crisis which your family has experienced recently. How did you cope?

3. Share practical ways in which couples can "pull together" and keep their relationship vibrant during extended periods of family stress.

# *Step 5*

## Prepare for the Golden Years

*By reaffirming their partnership and learning from the stress of their past, spouses can adapt to the changes of the empty nest and prepare for exciting, fruitful opportunities in their retirement.*

# 15

# *The Empty Nest*

Vonette and I were helping our youngest son, Brad, pack his car. He was leaving home—moving across the country to Washington D.C., to work for Senator William Armstrong from Colorado.

Just before he left, the three of us got down on our knees in the living room to pray. When we rose, he embraced each of us. My eyes misted as I silently thanked God for such a wonderful son.

As we walked outside, my mind wandered back to the first day I left him at boarding school . . .

First we had helped Zac, by this time a seasoned college student, settle into his dorm room at Life Bible College in Los Angeles. Then, a few days later, I flew with sixteen-year-old Brad to Stoneybrook, a Christian preparatory school in New York, where through the generosity of dear friends he was given a scholarship.

When the two of us arrived, we lugged his bags to his room. Later, I met the faculty and spoke at chapel.

When the time came for me to go, I could see that Brad was anxious to get settled and meet the rest of the boys. I felt unneeded. And lonely.

The thought of saying goodbye made my throat tighten. A flood of tears threatened to spill down my face. Wiping away the dampness, I hurriedly prepared to leave. I didn't want to embarrass him.

By the time I reached the car, my tears flowed in earnest, and in the privacy of the rental car I told the Lord how much I would miss him . . .

I felt the same ache in my throat now. As Brad drove away toward Washington, D.C., we waved valiantly. I forced a smile and stemmed my tears. *My little boy isn't little any more,* I thought as his car disappeared around a bend. *He's on his own now.*

And so were we. Zac had already left our nest and was soon to begin a family of his own, but I missed him just as much when he left.

I treasure these heartwarming memories of Zac and Brad. We'll always love our sons, and look forward to spending time with them whenever possible. But they are independent now. They don't need us like they did when they were young.

The empty nest stage of life can be the most exciting and creative time for couples. With the stress of child rearing only a memory, their marital relationship can grow deeper and richer. Even so, spouses face new challenges— those special stresses of the golden years.

## Preparing for the Golden Years

No matter how we approach life, we age. Feeling older, however, doesn't always match the number of years a person has lived.

The legendary baseball player Satchel Paige used to challenge, "How old would you be if you didn't know how old you was?" If we think we are ancient, we will be. But if we live creative and adventurous lives, we defy the stereotypes of old age.

How can we live a full life despite the pressures of aging? By preparing for the years ahead. And by utilizing the lessons we have learned from the stresses of our past.

This gives us a distinct advantage. Unlike a bride and groom setting out into the unfamiliar territory of marriage, we who reach the golden years have gained some wisdom from our many pressure-filled circumstances. We can use this wisdom to manage or reduce the stresses of our senior years, and thus enjoy happy, fruitful lives.

## Stress of the Empty Nest

The "empty nest syndrome" is a recent phenomenon created by increasing life expectancy. Before the medical advances of the 20th century, parents often did not survive long after their children left home. Today, however, many spouses live thirty to fifty years after their children are grown.

The empty nest brings with it a special set of stressors which can destroy a relationship. Many divorces occur at this period in the marriage cycle. This is so tragic, for these are the years when partners need each other for encouragement, comfort and care.

Let's look briefly at three of the major "golden age" stressors:

### 1. Loneliness

Without children in the home, a marital relationship undergoes radical change. Couples who have centered their lives around their children find the empty nest a particularly painful period of adjustment. Over the years, their marriage may have lost its vitality. They discover their relationship is merely a hollow shell, with nothing between them to prevent the loneliness.

## 2. Boredom

During this period, many spouses realize that their mate will never change those irritating habits nor conquer his weaknesses.

With children out of the nest, parents are forced into relating to each other. Spouses see their partner without the covering of parenthood. The only person to talk to at the dinner table is their mate. No energetic teenager livens their long evenings at home together. As a result, they find themselves wallowing in boredom and depression, resenting their bleak future and nurturing bad attitudes.

## 3. Painful Midlife Adjustments

Expectations and roles during the empty nest period change radically.

With her children gone, the wife is now free to pursue her occupation or ministry full time. She may enter the job force or a ministry area for the first time in many years, eager to attain the goals she has put off for so long.

At the same time, her husband has discovered his limitations in the work world. His career has become routine and dull. With his wife at work, he no longer feels the center of her attention. Her new excitement and awareness makes him realize how tired of the corporate rat-race he is. With occupational stress at a peak, he wants a change.

Thus, emotional stability is threatened. With no children at home for companionship and nurturing, the empty nest couple must reorganize their pattern of home life.

Yet the empty nest can be the beginning of a richer, fuller life. Many couples find profound satisfaction during this period. If they planned ahead, they have more financial resources and fewer expenses. They have fewer demands on their schedules. They have more time together and can concentrate fully on each other's company.

I encourage you to consider this time of life a gift from God to help you deepen your love for each other.

## Making the Transition Less Stressful

Vonette and I dedicated Zac and Brad to God before they were born. Our sons have belonged to Him all these years. We were just responsible to rear them in the love and fear of our Lord and to give them the best training we could.

Even so, that final break when they left our nest was hard to accept.

Perhaps you are about to enter this difficult period. Or you are already experiencing the empty nest. Let me share three important principles that will help make your transition to the empty nest less stressful.

### 1. Let Go

As our children grow into their teens and become mature adults, we must consciously give them back to God's care. Letting go is no easy task, as you may have discovered. Accepting the empty nest with a positive attitude in the power of the Holy Spirit helps to lessen the pain of separation.

As your nest empties, no doubt you will shed tears as did Vonette and I when we released Zac and Brad to independence. But as you let go, God can fill the void with exciting and fruitful new opportunities and relationships. We have found delight in pouring our lives into each other in order that we may be more effective in our ministry for our

Lord. We have also found more time to invest in the lives of many other young men and women and other adults as well.

## 2. Accept the Change

Sadly, many couples respond to the stress of an empty nest in the same negative way they learned to handle other critical situations. They try to keep the status quo.

We can, however, develop new strategies for adapting at any stage of life.

Instead of holding onto old patterns of living, embrace new ways of doing things. Cultivate an open, teachable spirit. Rebuild your empty home through the power of the Holy Spirit.

Recognize that both you and your partner have also changed over the years. Don't expect that "newlywed couple" to re-emerge after the children leave. Rather, begin reorganizing your relationship on the basis of who you are *now* instead of what you were years ago.

## 3. Adopt a Positive Attitude

Attitude makes all the difference in how couples adjust to the empty nest.

Self-pity and inflexibility only lengthen and aggravate a difficult transition. But a positive outlook opens our hearts and minds to the Lord's healing and helps ease the pain.

Vonette and I keep a positive attitude by welcoming the years ahead. We started alone, and once again we are enjoying "just the two of us." Though we believe the greatest investment we've made through the years is in the rearing of our sons, these present years in many ways are our most productive. We believe the best years of our lives are before us.

We urge you to taste the same joy. Rejoice in the partner God gave you. Plan to reap the benefits of your fruitful, godly life. Appreciate your life as it is. Look for the many positive results of growing older together.

## Developing a Fuller Life in the Empty Nest

Think of what's happening to older couples in our society. A greater number of wives are entering the job market at middle age, or even later. One mother-turned-grandmother, for example, became a nurse, specializing in pediatrics. More husbands are turning to a second career. We know a successful businessman who became a classroom teacher at forty-three.

You, too, can make the empty nest period an exciting and creative adventure. Let me share several practical suggestions to help you:

### 1. Step Into the Future

Using the empty nest as a stepping stone to the future prepares couples for many rewards later. Determine to live an active, purposeful life—as did a banker who entered seminary to prepare for ministry at age forty-seven; as did a friend who enrolled in graduate school to earn a degree in social work at age fifty-six.

I encourage you to decide which direction the Lord would have you take when your parenting days are over. Then use your extra time, money and concentration to set out on that path.

### 2. Expand Your Horizons

Living in an empty nest can be especially tedious if we have too narrow a focus. We must expand our horizons.

One way is to develop new ministries. One couple, for example, looked at their four-bedroom home and wondered what to do with all the space. Then they had an idea. Why not start weekend retreats?

Once a month, they invited ten people to their home on Friday evening through mid-day Saturday. They tried to include at least one person or couple who hadn't committed their lives to Jesus Christ. Guests could choose to sleep over or go back to their homes and return for breakfast. The group studied the Bible and prayed for each other during this time.

With a little imagination, you can think of other things to do. You could begin a ministry to international students. Or use your extra time for discipleship and evangelism. You may wish to travel to a part of the country you have never seen. Learn a new hobby or craft. Teach illiterate adults to read. Plant a garden. Whatever your activity, do something you have always wanted to do but couldn't while the children were at home, and do it for the glory of God.

Above all, keep growing. Use your creative abilities and adventurous spirit to improve your partnership.

### 3. Enrich Your Friendships

An effective way to reduce the stress of the empty nest is to dedicate your time to helping others. When you pour your life into someone else, the adjustments you make will be easier. The rapport and care you exchange with friends will soothe the lonely days.

### 4. Enjoy Life With Your Partner

Now Vonette and I view the empty nest as a second honeymoon. Joyful, abundant partnership means receiving our major rewards and strength from each other. It requires sharing our interests and time.

But what fun it is! We laughingly refer to this time of our lives as the "brighter years." And we are looking forward to the rest of our lives with great anticipation.

## For Reflection, Discussion and Action

1. What are you doing to prepare for the emptying of your nest? How will you make the transition less stressful?

2. What are the positive aspects of the empty nest?

3. There comes a time in every family when the parents must let go of their children. Think of ways to reduce the stress of letting your children go.

4. Take time with your partner to develop a strategy for making your empty nest years richer and fuller.

# 16

# *Growing in Retirement*

Dwight and Audrey Swanson were returning from their first trip as a retired couple. Dwight had completed an active forty-year career in business, most recently as CEO for Iowa Resources, Inc., a large, profitable utilities company based in Des Moines. They decided they were entitled to some leisure and time off. Then they wandered into a meeting held by Campus Crusade . . .

Ray and Burnette Whitehead's lives were full and productive. Ray was the founder and president of an engineering company. Burnette was involved in cultural and other activities with their children. At fifty-three, Ray decided to take an early retirement . . .

What do these couples have in common? Open to God's leading in their lives, they embarked on exciting new adventures during a time when other Christians are content to sit idle.

In recent years, Vonette and I have felt burdened for that strategic segment of society who possess a phenomenal, even revolutionary potential for serving

God — those sixty years and older. We envision many older couples serving Christ together in ways they never dreamed possible. We see them growing and learning through their retirement years, and using their talents and skills until the end of their lives.

## Preparing for Retirement

The stresses of the golden years defeat many Christian mates. Although we begin aging the moment we are born, often it isn't until our forties that we become aware of a gradual deterioration. As we move on in years, the rate of decline increases. No longer do experience and knowledge compensate for losses through aging. Couples we know who are in their young to middle years seem to look younger every year — a constant reminder that we have entered the last third of our lives.

Perhaps you are approaching retirement. What can you do to prepare for this stage of your life and reduce the stress of these twilight years? From our personal experiences, Vonette has these suggestions:

### 1. Accept Your Age

Did you know that Grandma Moses began oil painting at age seventy-five? And that she created her most famous work, *Christmas Eve,* at 101?

Or that Bach composed some of his best music at eighty-five? That Ronald Reagan became president of the United States, the most powerful and influential office in the secular world, at seventy and completed his second term of office at seventy-eight?

We could list many others who have made remarkable achievements in contributions to their fellow man in their golden years.

The Scriptures also record men and women who experienced and accomplished great things in their old age. Sarah and Abraham started a family well beyond child-rearing years. Joshua and Caleb led the Hebrew army across the Jordan to conquer the Promised Land when they were in their eighties.

The Lord regards the elderly with high honor.[1] Rejoice that He has given you so many years. Thank Him for every moment, each ability, and all the relationships you enjoy.

Do as Solomon urged and "rejoice in the wife of your youth."[2] Be grateful for every day you spend with your partner.

Face the reality of your situation. Don't futilely search for ways to keep yourself eternally young. Accept your limitations.

If you experience pain or loss as part of your aging process, live graciously day by day through the power of the Holy Spirit.

## 2. Make Peace With Life

To make peace with life, we must accept the certainty of our own death and that of our partner. When we realize that change is a part of God's loving plan for us, we can prepare for the sorrows we inevitably encounter. Put your mate's health and life in His hands. Ask God to strengthen your courage and bolster your hope, even as illness and death take their toll.

We have discovered that by flowing with the ups and downs of life in the power of the Holy Spirit, we can use the circumstances and stresses of the golden years to grow as a couple and to deepen our spiritual walk with the Lord.

## 3. Retrain for a Career With Fewer Physical Demands

Perhaps like Bill and me, you may not want to retire. You may wish to continue your present ministry or career long after most people have opted for the Gold Watch, Social Security and a rocking chair.

But what if you have no choice? What happens when your employer decides it's time for you to move on?

Even if you can continue your career, will you be physically up to it? Are you preparing for that event?

Choosing and training now for a career that you can handle in retirement is a wise decision if you plan to continue in the work force.

### 4. Prepare for a Loss of Income

Many senior citizens cannot maintain the salary or wages they earned in their fifties or early sixties. Retirement may mean going from two paychecks to none. You may find your resources stretched to the limit. What can you do to ease this problem? Here are a few ideas:

- Start a retirement fund early in your career.
- Set a budget before you quit work.
- Take care of major expenditures ahead of time, like replacing worn appliances or re-roofing your home.
- Reduce your debt.
- Keep saving and investing after you retire to help curb spending and slow the depletion of your reserve.
- Obtain counsel from a godly, competent financial advisor.

God controls events. No matter how much we plan, we have no assurance of a quiet, secure tomorrow. But our dependence on the Lord instead of our preparations will enable us to live fruitful, abundant lives through all our circumstances.

**5. Keep Active**

Our culture offers two views on aging.

One says that retirees should gradually pull away from former pursuits. Peace and contentment come only by withdrawing from an active role in society.

The other view holds that senior citizens must remain active at all costs. The elderly are not much different from middle-aged adults. Except for slowing down somewhat, older persons should work and participate in other activities as they once did.

Both views are valid when kept in balance. As we age, we will be progressively more limited in what we can do. Yet, if we listen and respond to God's voice, He will enable us to minister actively to the end of our lives.

## Living a Productive Life

Have you ever heard older Christians remark, "I've served the Lord for many years. Now it's time for me to sit back and let the younger people take over"?

God may change our ministry as we grow older, but He never asks us to retire from His work. At every age, we must be open to His calling.

Mrs. Erma Griswold, Bill's valued associate for more than twenty-five years, joined Campus Crusade at a time when most people stop working. But at sixty-seven, she was just getting started.

As a volunteer to our ministry, she has had a worldwide influence. She has lightened Bill's load tremendously and inspired all of our office staff by her faithful service.

At ninety-three, she is still a godly example of how productive the golden years can be.

Dwight and Audrey Swanson are another example.

Bill relates the story:

They had just taken their first trip as retirees. To end the month-long vacation, they stopped in Hershey, Pennsylvania, where Dwight had a speaking engagement at a utilities stockholders meeting.

While walking through the hotel, they discovered a musical group rehearsing for a Campus Crusade seminar and dinner that evening.

Since they had contributed to the ministry in the past, Dwight and Audrey decided to attend the seminar after he addressed the stockholders. At the end of the Campus Crusade meeting, they joined a reception line to greet us.

As we talked, I learned that Dwight had just retired from forty years in business.

"God sent you!" I exclaimed. "I've been praying for retired businessmen to provide our ministry with professional administrative help."

Although Dwight wasn't looking forward to assuming weighty responsibilities, he and Audrey visited Arrowhead Springs, where a short time later they decided to join this ministry.

For the first year, Dwight held the position of administrative associate. Then he became vice president of administration. His expertise in organizing people was invaluable.

Audrey joined the Campus Crusade Wives' Advisory Board. She worked with the Clothes Closet, a program to help fill the needs of Crusade staff facing a financial crisis or returning from overseas missions. She also became a prayer coordinator for Associates in Media, a Campus Crusade ministry in Hollywood.

Because of their availability, Dwight and Audrey gave

productive service beyond retirement, and their time with
Campus Crusade was rewarding and fruitful. Dwight continues to serve as chairman of the board of our International School of Theology.

God may not ask you to move across the country to be
a full-time volunteer in a Christian organization like Campus Crusade, but if you are available He will reveal ways in
which you can be fruitful for Him where you are. Keep yourself open to the Holy Spirit's leading, and He will direct you
to a fulfilling ministry.

I cannot think of a more rewarding ministry than
being an intercessor. As you have more free time, spend it
in the Lord's presence. Pray for your loved ones and friends
who have not yet received Christ as their Savior and Lord.
Intercede for your neighbors, your church, your pastor, a
missionary. Lift up our leaders in government. Claim 2
Chronicles 7:14 for our nation. Prayer for a revival to come
to our beloved land and a worldwide spiritual harvest.

I also encourage you to use your creative abilities and
talents to reach others for Christ. If there are children in
your neighborhood, adopt a "grandchild," loving and intro-
ducing him to God's love and forgiveness through Jesus
Christ. Or join the visitation team at your church.

Use your hobby as an opportunity to share Christ.
While teaching a knitting class or delivering homemade
meals to invalids, share your testimony of how God has
given you new life through Jesus Christ.

Live simply. Lay up your treasures in Heaven. Don't
invest all your resources in things of this world. When the
Lord Jesus Christ makes you aware of the needs of others,
be ready to help them. There is a law of God, as you sow
you reap. The more you help others, the more God will bless
and help you.

I urge you to step out in faith into new areas of Chris-

tian service. Don't let opportunities to share Christ and
minister to others in His name slip by during your golden
years.

Enjoying life is another secret to a productive retirement. If you start planning projects or volunteer work that
excites you before you retire, the transition can be uplift-
ing rather than depressing.

In addition to using your creative abilities and investing yourself in others, consider the little ways you could
make your life happier after you quit work. Sleep in a little later in the morning. Walk. Read those books you have
put off so long. Beautify your garden. Take time to enjoy
God's marvelous creation. Find exciting things to do with
your mate.

We have discovered that one of the greatest enjoy-
ments a couple can have during their golden years is
grandparenting. We love to play with our grandchildren,
take them places, tell them stories from our past, and listen to their chatter.

## The Fullness of the Golden Years

A wise counselor once told Job, "You shall live a long,
good life; like standing grain, you'll not be harvested until
it's time!"[3]

Ray and Burnette Whitehead are examples of this.

An early retirement was anything but the beginning
of a quiet life for them. When Ray left his contracting business at fifty-three to join our ministry, the busiest part of
his life began.

These years have taken them to two other continents
to live. For a year Ray put his business skills to work at our
headquarters, engineering and excavating for the village
conference center, amphitheater and office complex.

For six years, they lived in Latin America. Much of their time there was spent organizing evangelistic breakfasts and dinners for government and business leaders and their wives.

In 1974 they moved back to the United States and ministered to executives, helping them see how they could invest in God's work around the world. When our South African staff decided to start a similar ministry, Ray and Burnette took a group of executives from the United States to participate in South Africa's first Executive Seminar.

After leading a few more tours to Africa, this dedicated couple moved to South Africa in 1979. Their primary aim was to minister to the black leaders of South Africa's Black Homelands. With three special assets—his white hair, his nationality and his boldness—Ray befriended and ministered to many who had not been reached for Christ.

"As long as I'm physically able," Ray affirms, "I'll never be satisfied unless I'm right in the thick of the battle. I could have made a lot of money if I'd kept working. But if God can use me to see one soul turn to Him, it's worth all that. We don't have a lot of money, but we've never lived so well—or been so happy and content."[4]

How about you? Are you experiencing what they have discovered? That the later years truly are golden as ripened grain? We urge you to dedicate your entire life and marriage to the service of our gracious Savior, Jesus Christ.

Whatever circumstances or stage of life you find yourself in right now, remember that your partnership is the most secure asset you have to manage tension and grow through the pressures of a busy lifestyle.

Vonette and I encourage you to use the five steps we have shared in this book to deepen your relationship. To summarize, these steps were:

1. Enter into a partnership with your spouse to provide a secure foundation to handle change and pressure.

2. Establish God-centered priorities to give your relationship direction and control through the storms of life.

3. Use praise, communication and your sex life to reduce the stress of daily living.

4. Accept your children as God's plan for your childrearing years to ease the tension of parenting.

5. Reaffirm your partnership, and use the lessons you have learned in life to prepare for your golden years.

By following these steps, you will experience the immeasurable joy and richness of a marriage dedicated to the Lord and to each other. With God at the helm, you will conquer the angry waves of crisis and enjoy beautiful sunsets together in the midst of turmoil. You will know the satisfaction of a fulfilling, vibrant, fruitful relationship that comes from growing through the stresses in marriage.

## For Reflection, Discussion and Action

1. Several biblical characters were mentioned in this chapter as examples of people who were used by God in their elder years. With your mate, select one of them and do a character study of his life and ministry.

2. If you knew that you were going to retire in a year, what specific plans for your retirement would you be making now?

3. With your mate, think of ways that God can use you

for His glory in your golden years. Invite the Holy
Spirit to give you creative ideas.

# Part 3

# A
# Personal Word

# 17

# *Building a Home in a Pull-Apart World*

## A Word to Women From Vonette

The move of our international headquarters to Arrowhead Springs took me away from an active campus ministry, from our church where we were established and involved, and away from long time friends.

At first, I assisted in establishing the conference center, aided in beginning the lay ministry, and helped write Crusade training materials. All of this was exciting and I loved being involved with Bill, though it was different from what we had known on the campus.

As the ministry grew, God brought us qualified people who were able to assume responsibility for some of the areas in which I had been involved.

Although I loved being at home more and having time of my own to manage, I found myself frustrated at times by a lack of challenge. I didn't feel as productive and personally involved in Bill's activities as I had once been.

In conversations with Bill, I would often express my concern and ask what he thought I should do.

One day he put his arms around me tenderly and said, "Honey, if you can just keep our home running smoothly while our sons are young, you can be of most help to me. I understand there are many other things you could be doing. But right now the boys and I need you in our home."

Although Bill and the children occupied the highest place in my life after the Lord, my diminished involvement in the ministry was still threatening to my sense of significance. Even as I struggled with the transition, I realized that having committed my life to Christ, knowing Bill loved me, knowing I was contributing to our personal and ministry goals, was enough. I joyfully decided to fit in where Bill needed me, a decision I never regretted.

My willingness to fit in where most needed for our family's sake enabled Bill to function more effectively as president of our rapidly expanding organization and allowed me to enjoy the fuller privileges of motherhood and homemaking. I began to pour my energies more into our children's activities, the PTA and our church.

Undoubtedly every career woman faces the temptation to put her family in second place. I could have easily done that. The question we all ask is, "How can I make a maximum long-range contribution to making the world a better place in which to live for the glory of God?" Or in my case, "How do we build a secure, loving home in a pull-apart world?"

## Women Can Make a Difference

Recently I spoke at a New England area conference for women students from Smith, Radcliff, Mount Holyoke, MIT, Yale, Harvard, Dartmouth, Brown and other universities. The message I shared with them was that the influence and impact of their lives and other women like them will determine what life will be like on this planet in the 21st century.

"Today's woman," writes Elizabeth Skoglund, a contemporary author, "has potential for growth, opportunity for equality, and a choice of roles. She can compete with pride in the marketplace, and she can, with equal dignity, stay at home and raise children. Or, she can do both. Above all, she can still be a woman, no matter what her role."[1]

Proverbs 31 describes one model of Christian womanhood. I appreciate the way one unidentified writer has paraphrased her characteristics:

- She faithfully satisfies and supports her husband, a respected leader in the community.
- She purchases supplies from distant sources.
- She provides food and beautiful clothing for her household.
- She directs and manages the household servants.
- She invests in real estate and engages in commercial agriculture, financed by her own earnings.
- She trades for profit and does charitable work.
- She teaches wisely, diligently cares for her children, and administrates the affairs of her household.

What a woman!

Now before you panic, let me say that God doesn't want you to run a ten-ring circus; He doesn't require you to pursue the lifestyle of the Proverbs woman. She is an example of what God allows a woman to be—if she so chooses.

God does not view the fair sex as second-rate men but as unique individuals with almost unlimited capabilities.

So the question is not, "Can I experience my full potential and lead or influence my world as a Christian?" but "What kind of influence am I going to have and what will determine the choices I make?" As women, we *will* have an influence. We must make sure that our lives serve as positive, constructive and eternal examples.

I believe the most rewarding, sustaining lifestyle is one rooted in a personal, trusting relationship with Jesus Christ, characterized by obedience to the way of life He desires. We experience this as we place the full weight of our identity not on what we are, but on the One who will never change.

Women significantly determine the moral standards of a nation. Writing of the United States in the early 1800s, De Tocqueville stated in *Democracy in America,* "Now as I come to the end of this book in which I have recorded so many considerable achievements of the Americans, if anyone asks me what I think was the chief cause of the extraordinary prosperity and the growing power of this nation, I should answer that it is due to the superiority of her women."

Consequently, we have an awesome responsibility to use our talents and gifts to make a difference in our homes, in our communities and in our nation.

## Building a Godly Home

The Proverbs 31 woman, however, achieves her greatest influence in her home. Her first priority is to the needs of her loved ones. Although she works outside the home, she gives her foremost attention to the needs of her husband and children. She is a marvelous, realistic model of how we, too, can build a godly home in the midst of a pull-apart world. Here are several key principles which she exemplifies:

## 1. Fear God

*"A woman who fears and reverences God shall be greatly praised."*[2]

Usually the woman sets the atmosphere and pace in the home. She may either establish a calm, loving mood or a hectic, disagreeable one. If she neglects her spiritual walk, her family suffers. But if she depends on the Holy Spirit, she creates a place where everyone feels comfortable and secure.

Let me encourage you to feast on the Word of God daily to refresh your spirit and keep your moods gentle and loving. Fill your home with the sound of recorded Scripture, Christian songs and hymns. This will help you establish an environment in which you can settle squabbles, discipline children and soothe hurt feelings with the mercy and justice that only God can give you.

Many men will not compete for spiritual headship and will bow out if their wives insist on taking the spiritual leadership role. If your husband accepts his God-given role as the priest and servant-leader of his home, encourage his efforts and help him gain confidence in his leadership.

But what happens if your husband's job frequently takes him away from home? Or if he neglects or refuses to serve as the priest in your family? Should you assume the spiritual leadership?

Yes. Accept the responsibility as if he had delegated it to you. Gently and lovingly encourage him in his relationship with God. More important, pray constantly for him and trust the Lord to enable him to accept his God-given responsibility in the home.

Keep in mind that one purpose of the home is to rear children in the fear of the Lord to have character, integrity and purpose. This will enable them to take their God-given place on the world scene as responsible and accountable citizens and leaders in helping to build a better world.

## 2. Make Your Home a Priority

*"She watches carefully all that goes on throughout her household, and is never lazy."*[3]

No institution is more important than the home. An atmosphere of love, loyalty and caring can best be maintained within the family circle. Self-esteem and acceptance flourish like well-watered plants. Through our families we build the church and our nation.

Yet this world tells us that wifely duties rank below many other activities. The secular community wants us to believe that cooking, cleaning, wiping runny noses and changing diapers do not have the dressing of success.

These pressures are why a wife must make sure her home is top priority. I regard my responsibilities as wife and mother a privilege and the highest calling.

The daughter of our dear friend Mrs. Louis Evans Sr. told me a story about her mother. When she was a young girl, she came home to find her mother sitting on the back steps, head in her hands, exhausted. The daughter noticed a long line of freshly-beaten rugs on the clothesline.

"Oh, Mother," she lamented as she sat beside her, "I am so sorry you have to work so hard. You could have been a great musician or a wonderful teacher. But here you are a housewife."

At her words, Mrs. Evans picked herself up proudly. "My dear, I am *not* the wife of a house. I am building a home. And that takes a lot of beating rugs, washing dishes and caring for children."

Many times over the years, however, the pulls of the outside world threatened to distort my focus. I have had to continually reassess my priorities. I frequently stopped to find out the needs of my family and how I could meet them.

I tried to balance the time I spent with each person.

Physical arrangements sometimes posed special challenges. When will I clean my house? Do I have time for the laundry? Or am I so wrapped up in minor housekeeping details that I'm neglecting my family's emotional needs? Or opportunities to minister to others? All these concerns required constant evaluation.

A dedicated wife, I have learned, daily commits herself to the task of building a godly home. She cannot afford to let others shoulder her responsibility. That doesn't mean that she can't get support from outside the home. But she sees to the welfare of each member personally.

### 3. Reach Out to Others Through Your Home

*"She sows for the poor, and generously gives to the needy."*[4]

The Scriptures give many examples of women who used their homes for ministry—the poor widow, who fed and housed Elijah; Naomi, who took in her daughter-in-law, Ruth; Priscilla, who opened her home to the apostle Paul on his missionary journey.

Bill's mother, Mary Lee, was a modern example of the Proverbs 31 woman. She was a well-educated, fine-fibered person, a former teacher who enjoyed classic literature and cherished her Bible. She married a cattle rancher and gave birth to eight children. Although life on the ranch was not easy in rural America at that time, she lived an attractive Christian life before her family and friends and never complained or criticized another person. She made her home a haven for the family and was always available to care for neighbors in need. Her home was so popular that she often did not know how many would be present for a meal.

When anyone in the community mentioned the most godly person they knew, Mrs. Bright's name usually came up first. Her influence is still felt around the world through her family.

I encourage you to enlist your family's creativity to make your home a center for evangelism and caring. Entertain non-Christian friends, or lead an evangelistic coffee for women. Build friendships with neighbors and share Jesus Christ with them.

Why not celebrate Christmas with a birthday party for Jesus and invite your children's playmates? Bible clubs for children in your backyard present an excellent opportunity as well.

Plan a picnic with a non-Christian family. Encourage your husband and children to pray for each guest ahead of time. Help your family care for the needs of your visitors and share their testimonies with someone during the outing.

## Helping Your Husband Succeed as a Leader

The Proverbs 31 woman helped her husband succeed.[5] He trusted her because of her unselfish attitudes and actions. Would you like to know how to encourage your husband to reach his full potential, despite the pressures of his hectic life? Let me give you four suggestions:

### 1. Intercede for Him

Bringing your husband's needs and stresses before the Lord is the greatest service you can do for him.

I keep a prayer diary. Of course, Bill heads the top of the list. I put down specific prayer requests, asking the Lord to give him discernment in the decisions he must make. I pray for his spiritual walk, his physical health and the influence others have on him and that he has on those around him.

Often, he will mention a situation of concern. Sometimes he asks me to pray for him at a certain time of the day. I bring these matters to the Lord, then ask later about the results.

Whatever method you use to pray for your husband, be consistent and faithful. Thank the Lord for the growth and maturity you see in his life. And for the contribution he makes to you and your home.

## 2. Support His Leadership

There can be only one head in a marriage partnership. God ordained that position for the husband. Napoleon said he would rather have one weak commander than two strong ones who were constantly competing. There should never be any strife for supremacy in the marriage partnership. The apostle Paul writes:

> Wives, submit to your husband as to the Lord. For the husband is the head of the wife as Christ is head of the church. Now as the church submits to Christ, so also wives should submit to their husbands in everything.[6]

The apostle gives this direction after first admonishing, "Honor Christ by submitting to each other."[7] Paul leaves no doubt, however, as to who should have the final authority. And he makes it clear that the wife should voluntarily follow her husband's leadership in all areas. That does not mean she blindly follows or has no input to where that leadership will lead. The wise husband who "loves his wife as Christ loved the church" will consult and work toward agreement.

From the beginning of our marriage, I found it easy to support and promote my husband because he knew where he was going. He had vision. He had courage. He had faith. And he was willing to take risks for the Lord. I was eager to make a contribution to his life and ministry. As a result, I looked for ways in which I could complement and be an encouragement to him. I sought his advice and his direction, checking to make sure I was doing what he needed most.

The apostle Peter describes a wife's submission to her husband as beautiful.[8] Proverbs 31:11 praises the noble wife because she is one who richly satisfies her husband's needs. She supplies that which no one else can.

Yet some women feel that this role as a homemaker is demeaning and makes her inferior and less significant. But Jesus explained,

> Whosoever wishes to become great among you shall be your servant, and whoever wishes to be first among you shall be your slave; just as the Son of Man did not come to be served, but to serve, and to give His life a ransom for many.[9]

Bill often says that the three greatest influences in his life have been women: his mother, me, and Dr. Henrietta Mears. Women have the greatest opportunity as wives and mothers to fulfill that Scripture and follow our Lord's example.

One of the essential ingredients of being supportive in submission is adapting. We need to fit in with our husbands' plans and schedule.

Rather than trying to make our husbands conform to us, we should help maximize their potential, enabling them to be all they possibly can be.

Wives, if we don't adapt, we put a tremendous strain on our marriage. We cause our husbands either to abandon their leadership roles or to rigidly enforce rules. Our lack of conformity to God's order in the family weakens our partnership.

Consider submission a trust from God. Remember that supporting your husband is obedience to your heavenly Father also.

### 3. Respect Him

Have you ever watched a wife who outwardly submits to her husband but inwardly holds him in contempt? She effectively destroys their marital intimacy and undermines his self-esteem.

If we understand the differences between men and women, we will recognize the importance of treating our husbands with deep respect. Generally, women need love and security for fulfillment while men seek after significance and recognition. Respect is one way a husband achieves significance.

You may say, "I cannot respect my husband."

Then praise and affirm your husband in the areas in which he excels. Help him with his weaknesses in a non-threatening, confidential manner. Support him in what he feels God has called him to do.

When Bill stepped out in faith to buy Arrowhead Springs, many people felt he was making a grave mistake. One friend, one of our major financial supporters, strongly opposed our purchasing Arrowhead and kept expecting the project to fail. When Bill didn't agree with him, the friend warned, "If you buy this property, I won't give any more money to the ministry." He was faithful to his word.

He took me aside one day. "Don't worry, Vonette," he said calmly. "I've set aside a large sum of money to take care of you and Bill and the ministry when this thing falls through and he falls flat on his face."

Although my faith was shaky, I supported my husband and assured our friend, "God will supply our needs."

Of course, the Lord did meet our needs day by day, month by month until the miracle of Arrowhead Springs was complete and our final payment was made. Through the years since the purchase of Arrowhead Springs in 1962, hundreds of thousands of people from all over the world have received training in discipleship and evangelism here.

In the meantime, I learned a valuable lesson. Although in private I may question or disagree with Bill, publically I always support him when he believes God is leading him to undertake a special project. I choose to put aside our differences to work beside him. That is one way I can show how much I respect and believe in him.

Be sensitive to how you can increase your husband's stature among his friends and co-workers. When he feels discouraged, help him stick to the course he has set. Don't make mountains out of molehills if he displays poor judgment.

## 4. Listen to Him

Men need their wives to listen to them.

A few years ago, I began doing a lot of needlepoint. After completing four or five pieces, I started on a large project. As I was finishing, Bill asked, "You aren't going to do *more* needlepoint, are you?"

"Why would you say that?" I asked, surprised.

"It seems to me that you could be doing something more important with your time."

His comment made me analyze the situation. At every opportunity, I would concentrate on my needlepoint, usually on an airplane. As I sewed, I would listen to a tape and get lost in my thoughts while Bill read. We weren't talking as much. Soon after I completed that project, I put away my sewing and began listening to him and he to me.

As involved as I am, I have to make time to listen. No matter what the demands of my work, when Bill needs my attention, he comes first. I may have to ask him to delay his conversation until later, but I honor his request.

Take the time to let your husband share what is on his mind and heart. He may express his thoughts factually rather than emotionally, but give him an opportunity to tell you about his failures and discouragements without criticism. Express your admiration for his successes. Build his trust by keeping his confidences. It may be necessary to set specific times to talk, then give him your undivided attention.

## Building Bridges Between Family and Career

One of the major challenges faced by today's two-career families is achieving balance. We *do* live in a pull-apart world where the demands of the work environment destroy the unity in the home. But you can minimize the effects of this pressure by maintaining a positive attitude toward your career, enlisting the cooperation of your family, and inviting your family to participate in decision making.

To keep a positive attitude toward the demands of your career, remind yourself of the fulfillment and rewards of your work.

Involve your family in your professional life. Describe your work duties and talk about the people you see at your office. Take your husband and children on a tour of the workplace.

Help them to see the advantages of your career. Explain the financial blessings and the necessity of the extra income. Talk about the importance of developing your skills and abilities, and show them how your job contributes to their own growth and independence.

Enlist the cooperation of your family by inviting them to share in the daily chores. The scrambled eggs may taste rubbery when your teenage son cooks, but learn to appreciate his efforts anyway.

If your daughter misses more spots than she cleans when washing the floor, use the opportunity to teach her how to do a thorough job. Be willing to lower your standards a little when your preschooler straightens his room.

Avoid criticism. Many wives sabotage their efforts to gain cooperation by never being satisfied with the results. Instead, praise your husband and children when they help.

Gently correct your children when they intentionally do an unsatisfactory job. Recognize the difference between laziness and a lack of maturity to handle the responsibility. Expecting too much of a child before he is mature enough to accomplish what is expected will only frustrate him.

Family participation in decision making is a vital span on the bridge between family and career. Have you ever noticed how much harder a person works if he is involved in the decision making? Or how he drags his feet if someone imposes a job on him? Sometimes women make important decisions that affect their families without discussing them.

If you are planning a party in your home, for example, discuss your plans with the whole family—first. You can imagine how much more enthusiastically everyone would respond.

Consider your family a team. Encourage them to use their gifts, talents and personalities to help you ease the pressure of too little time and too many jobs. Of course, there will still be moments when you will have to insist firmly that your family help. But with your positive encouragement, they will be more likely to feel that their contribution to family life is valuable and desired.

I encourage you to make your home the center of your attention, even though you live a busy lifestyle. Use your talents to create a nest where each person can stretch and grow in a cradle of security. The result will be a unified group that can more effectively manage the stresses of living in a fast-paced world.

Don't be discouraged if you can't make the change all at once. Change requires time, commitment and maturity. But in this world of turmoil, the rewards for providing a stable, loving, Christ-centered home cannot be equaled.

With time, we can become more like the godly woman of Proverbs 31 who is "a woman of strength and dignity."[10] And the results of our dedication?

> Her children stand and bless her; so does her husband. He praises her with these words: "There are many fine women in the world, but you are the best of them all!"[11]

Who could ask for higher praise and satisfaction in building a home in a pull-apart world?

## For Reflection, Discussion and Action

1. List several women who have influenced your life for good. How did their examples inspire you?

2. How can you make your home a priority and still reach out to others? Implement at least one of these ideas this week.

3. In what ways are you helping your husband succeed as a leader? What additional things can you do to strengthen his potential as a leader?

# 18

# *Radical Lover— Intimate Leader*

## *A Word to Men From Bill*

A Japanese magazine has a picture of a butterfly on one of its pages. Its wings are a dull gray until warmed by one's hand. The touch causes the special inks in the printing to react, and the butterfly is transformed into a rainbow of color.

Throughout this book, Vonette and I have shared many principles that will help you transform your marriage into a rainbow of beauty. At this point you may wonder, "Where do I begin?"

Everything we have said hinges upon one basic premise in God's Word:

> Husbands, love your wives just as Christ loved the church and gave himself up for her."[1]

What does it mean to love as Christ loved the church? Why is this love so crucial?

Every Christian husband knows he should love his wife. But few really understand that it takes a radical kind of love to have a truly healthy, happy marriage.

Loving as Christ loves *is* radical. Picture it this way: Radical love is a finely cut diamond with many sparkling facets. Let's consider four of these qualities for a moment.

## 1. Radical Love Is Sacrificial

Unlike the Hollywood image of love which is based on lust and selfishness, Christ's love is rooted in selflessness and sacrifice. The apostle Paul's words to the Ephesians provide the key to this principle: Christ *gave himself up* for the church. Sacrificial love cost our Savior His life on the cross.

Likewise, Christ's love calls upon us to make sacrifices, to yield our rights and preferences for the sake of our wife. To lay aside our personal desires and ambitions for those of our spouse. To love sincerely and purely, with cordial and ardent affection. To cherish without reservation regardless of our partner's imperfections and failures.

We cannot love sacrificially in our own strength. By nature, we are jealous, envious and boastful. We are proud, haughty, selfish and demand our own way. But God puts His love into our hearts by the Holy Spirit the moment we receive Jesus Christ into our lives.

How long has it been since you showed sacrificial love to your wife? Take a moment, right now, to reflect on this question. Think of ways you can "give yourself up" to your wife. Make a list. Then ask God by faith to help you love her sacrificially as Christ loves the church.

## 2. Radical Love Takes the Initiative

Christ's sacrificial love can take a strife-torn marriage and transform it into a beautiful, rich relationship. Perhaps you are thinking, "But you don't know *my* wife. She's impossible! When she changes her attitude, I'll change mine!"

Radical love, however, is aggressive. It takes the initiative. It follows God's precept of "first love."[2] It reaches out in reconciliation when she is least deserving.

With the purest and deepest kind of love, our Lord modeled this principle. He took the initiative to reconcile us while we were yet in sin. Paul said, ". . . But God showed his great love for us by sending Christ to die for us while we were still sinners."[3]

The Greek word used in the Scriptures to describe this love is *agape*. It is expressed not through mere emotions, but as an act of one's will. We must not wait to *feel* loving before taking the initiative. We must choose to love by *faith*.

When Jesus sacrificed Himself on the cross for our sins, He did so by faith that we would respond to His redeeming love. He didn't wait until we were good; He loved first. This is what our Lord's "first love" principle means.

If you and your wife are experiencing conflict, I encourage you to begin loving her by faith. Take the first step in reconciliation. Ask the Holy Spirit to fill you with His power and Christ's radical love. Then pray for her. Talk to her. Show concern for her needs. And watch God work through you to calm the storm.

### 3. Radical Love Is Considerate

Many couples suffer needless turmoil because the husband is inconsiderate of his wife. Vonette and I are no exception.

She is strong and shares her opinions freely, and I always know where she stands on issues. I like her that way. Her sensitivities and abilities complement mine, and in many instances she has helped me see how to better solve a problem. But in the early years of our marriage, I didn't always appreciate her way of thinking.

If she disagreed with a decision I had made, I saw her as a deterrent to my plans and felt threatened. I had made up my mind and that was that! And instead of discussing the problem, I often walked out of the house.

The apostle Peter admonishes, "Husbands . . . be considerate as you live with your wives, and treat them with respect as the weaker partner and as heirs with you of the gracious gift of life, so that nothing will hinder your prayers."[4]

Being considerate, I have discovered, means treating Vonette with respect and valuing her opinions. Over the years, I have learned to talk about our differences and be more considerate of her needs and understanding of her temperament. I have realized that the Lord often speaks through her, so when we disagree I listen to her viewpoint.

And I no longer head for the nearest door.

Sometimes it's the little things that count most in being considerate of our wives. Like coming home from the office on time when Vonette has taken precious moments to prepare me a delicious meal.

Then there's picking up after myself. The last thing Vonette wants to do is clean up my mess at home after she's put in a hard day at the office or just before guests arrive.

Going shopping with your wife also shows consideration.

One evening when I was almost buried behind a stack of "urgent" reading materials and dictations, Vonette needed to go to the grocery store.

"Do you have time to go with me?" she asked.

Grocery shopping wasn't exactly what I had in mind for my evening. But I don't like Vonette going out alone after dark.

I laughed. "It'll be a sacrifice and a tremendous challenge to my future, but I will."

I'm like a kid in a candy store when it comes to grocery shopping. As we strolled the aisles, I kept throwing items into our cart. I spotted all kinds of bargains—and diet food. I even grabbed a can opener on sale.

By the time we reached the check-out counter, we looked like a couple buying groceries for a huge family. Our bill was considerably higher than when Vonette shops alone.

But she loves it when I go with her. Shopping turns into a safari, stalking groceries in a forest of shelves. And we come home with a carfull of bagged prey.

Taking interest in projects around the house is another way to be considerate.

In 1984 we decided to redecorate our house. The carpets had grown threadbare and the sofas needed recovering. We had entertained approximately 60,000 guests for dinners, luncheons and receptions since the house had last been decorated. And because of limited funds, we had put off redecorating for a long time.

One day a staff member said very kindly, "Bill, your home is the 'White House' of this ministry. If you don't have the money to redecorate it, I will." I got the message.

Together we began making our selections of decor and color. We readily agreed on most of our choices, but the living room was not pulling together.

I like blue. If I had my way, it would be the dominant color throughout the house, particularly in the living room. But Vonette wasn't excited about my choice so we kept working at our selection until we both were happy.

She sought the advice of a decorator friend, who suggested a color scheme of coral with light blue accents. Vonette was sure I would never accept that.

Of course, I try to impress her that my taste in decorating is better than hers! But actually her preference usually is best. I took one look at the decorator's suggestion and exclaimed, "That's it! Vonette looks great in coral. Let's wrap the living room around her."

The coral color pulled the blue decor together beautifully and we were both happy with the result.

I'm sure you can think of many other ways to be considerate. Take a few moments, right now, to jot down your ideas. Be creative. Ask God to help you. Showing consideration to your wife, even the smallest amount, will go a long way toward reducing the tensions in your marriage.

### 4. Radical Love Encourages Development

A considerate husband will always encourage his wife to develop spiritually, personally, socially and vocationally.

During a question-and-answer session, a young man expressed his concern that many single women who are involved in ministry are not interested in marriage for fear they will lose their significance in ministry.

I replied, "I don't blame them. If a man desires a wife to be only his housekeeper, laundress and cook, what woman would want to sacrifice serving the Lord in a significant ministry for such an unrewarding role?"

A man who wishes to make a woman his partner will realize that they can achieve more together than either could do separately. A woman will respond to partnership and look upon that kind of relationship as a significant ministry and lifestyle.

Many of us were reared to be "macho men." A husband and father was the lord of his kingdom and he expected his wife and children to bow to his every demand. Quite a contrast to the example of our dear Lord as described in Philippians:

> Your attitude should be the kind that was shown us by Jesus Christ, who, though he was God, did not demand and cling to his rights as God, but laid aside his mighty power and glory, taking the disguise of a slave and becoming like men. And he humbled himself even further going so far as actually to die a criminal's death on a cross.[5]

The only way to love as Christ did is to walk in the power of the Holy Spirit moment by moment as He did. Only He can enable you to have that supernatural, unconditional and unshakable love for your wife.

I encourage you to lay aside your personal desires and ambitions to meet her needs as Christ did for us. Love without reservation or expecting anything in return. Pour your life into hers. Be sensitive to her. Consult her and respect her judgment. Keep her informed on the issues that concern you. Then follow through with your actions.

## Intimate Leader

Why is loving our wives as Christ loved the church so crucial? Because our Lord commands it and because out of radical love emerges intimate leadership.

Next to his relationship to the Lord, an intimate leader is one who sees ministering to his wife as his highest calling in life.

Our first priority in this calling is to model spiritual leadership. A godly husband realizes that he shows through his example how the heavenly Father relates to His children. So this man takes seriously the biblical admonition to be "head of the wife as Christ is the head of the church."[6]

As high priest in his home, he prepares himself for leadership through consistent Bible study and prayer. He understands his accountability before God to nurture his wife in her walk with the Lord. Following the example of our Lord, he leads her with gentleness and consideration and never finds it necessary to demand submission. His character and example inspire cooperation and trust.

He creates an environment of warmth and intimacy by sharing himself with her, by placing her hurts and desires before his own, and by pleasing her in the little things of life.

Does this sound like an impossible journey? None of us can expect to achieve intimate leadership with sinless perfection. But we can rely on the power of the Holy Spirit to transform us into men of God, enabling us to love by faith.

An intimate leader also takes the lead in evangelism.

I am convinced by the examples and teachings of the Lord Jesus and the church of the New Testament that every Christian must be an aggressive witness for Christ and help fulfill the Great Commission as our Lord commanded.[7] The duty of every intimate leader is to inspire his wife and children by example and deed to obey this command.

When Vonette and I moved into our home in Bel Air three minutes from the UCLA campus, I was excited about how we could use it for our ministry. The first day we lived in that house, I spoke to a group of men at one of the fraternities. After the meeting, a young man followed me home for counsel and was the first to receive Christ in our house. Eventually, many hundreds of students experienced their first moments of new birth within those walls.

The best place to model our passion for lost souls is at home. Ministry to others in the core of family life teaches each member how to share Christ's love and forgiveness.

## Building Intimate Leadership
## Through Radical Love

Radical love, we have seen, finds its expression in sacrifice. It takes the initiative with reconciliation. It considers others before itself. But intimate leadership embraces yet another dimension.

Service.

Christ's example was clear. He came to serve. The Gospel of Mark records:

> Whoever wants to become great among you must be your servant, and whoever wants to be first must be slave of all. For even the Son of Man did not come to be served, but to serve, and to give his life as a ransom for many."[8]

Our Lord's disciples had great difficulty with this precept. At the Last Supper, they argued among themselves over who would be the greatest in the kingdom of God. Jesus corrected them lovingly:

> In this world the kings and great men order their slaves around, and the slaves have no choice but to like it! But among you, the one who serves you best will be your leader."[9]

Godly principles often seem paradoxical. To receive, we must give away. To live, we must die. To be exalted, we must be humble. To harvest, we must sow. To lead, we must serve.

The principle of servanthood is in sharp contrast to how many husbands see themselves.

Someone once said that husbands and wives are often like boiled potatoes sitting side by side on the same platter. What they need is a "heavenly masher" to come down and make them truly one. Unfortunately, many men see *themselves* as heavenly mashers. They rule their households as though they were iron-fisted dictators. "I'm boss here!" they declare. "And you do what I say, when I say, and how I say." These husbands violate Christ's example of servanthood, love and leadership and stand in the way of the Holy Spirit's work in their home.

During the Last Supper, Jesus began to wash the disciples' feet. When He came to Peter, Peter waved Him off. "Master, you shouldn't be washing our feet like this!"

Our Lord's answer is just as relevant today. "But if I don't, you can't be my partner."

Humility, Jesus was saying, is the key to a servant's heart. Without it, we cannot be partners with Him in intimate leadership.

I love Peter's response. "Then wash my hands and head as well—not just my feet."[10]

In other words, "Bathe me completely in Your humility, Lord. I want to be like You."

Let this be your prayer, too. Ask God to wash you thoroughly in our Lord's humility that you may be a partner with Him in leading your family. And seek to walk daily in that humility as you follow God's plan for leadership in your home.

## Following God's Plan

Many families experience turmoil because the husband doesn't take his proper role as a servant leader. No husband can afford to neglect his godly responsibility. Leading your wife by our Lord's tender mercies will help you build a vibrant, exciting, harmonious relationship.

I strongly urge you to keep *your* leadership on track. And to take the necessary steps to fulfill your God-given role as a radical lover and intimate leader.

## For Reflection, Discussion and Action

1.  Review the three qualities of radical love. How can you demonstrate these qualities in your relationship with your wife?

2.  What does it mean to love one's wife "as Christ loved the church?" Name practical ways that you as a husband can love your wife in this manner.

3.  What is the secret to building intimate leadership? How are you applying this principle in your relationship? In what ways can you improve?

# 19

# *The World Awaits*

You now know that the Brights live in an atmosphere of stress and that we have had to develop ways of dealing with it on a continuing basis. The lessons we have shared with you were not learned quickly; they were hammered out on the anvil of many years of experience.

Contrary to what the world would have us believe, the Christian does not have to experience conflict to be normal. Disagreements, yes. But these, we have found, can be resolved in an open, rational way through discussion and mutual submission — even though they may have deep emotional roots.

From early in our marriage, we believed that God had called us as a couple to help change the world. He has been real to both of us. We love the Lord Jesus Christ with all our hearts and are enthusiastic about sharing our faith with others. We are still excited about the vision which God gave us and the projects we have endeavored to accomplish. It is a source of great joy to think that our lives together can make a difference in the world for the glory of God.

Thus we have always considered the cause to which we have given our lives so much more important than the stress created by the atmosphere in which we live. Because of this, we have been able to focus on the positive benefits of our calling and therefore we do not usually feel burdened by the stress of the moment.

Don't think that you have to emulate our lifestyle. God wants to be original with each of us. We have simply made ourselves available to the Lord and responded to His particular call for our lives.

We believe that the basic principles we have discovered can, under the guidance and enabling of the Holy Spirit, help you work out your own responses to the stress that you are experiencing.

Being filled with the Spirit, using the Throne Check, and developing a contract that expresses your commitment to our Lord and to each other are practical ways you can meet the pressures of the future. As you maintain your first love for Christ and invite the Holy Spirit to control and empower you, you can meet the many demands you face daily.

There's a world to be reached for Jesus Christ. The biblical values that have governed our society for the past two hundred years, particularly in the United States, are eroding rapidly. The Christian lifestyle is increasingly being viewed as outmoded. The biblical worldview is not understood, even in many so-called Christian homes. But God is calling individuals and couples to a radical commitment to make themselves available to share His love and forgiveness in the most positive and effective manner.

God promises us victory, and most assuredly a life of genuine significance and personal fulfillment, as we respond to His call to help fulfill the Great Commission in our generation.

The last forty years have been an exciting adventure

as we have chosen to obey God's call upon our lives. As a result, we have experienced and continue to experience the reality of God's promise in Ephesians 3:20: "Glory be to God who by his mighty power at work within us is able to do far more than we would ever dare to ask or even dream of — infinitely beyond our highest prayers, desires, thoughts, or hopes" (TLB). The blessings of God on our lives, our marriage, and our family have far exceeded our greatest expectations.

The world is waiting for the impact of your life. We invite you to come help change this world.

# NOTES

### Chapter 1: The Uninvited Guest
1. Matthew 11:28-30.

### Chapter 2: The Many Faces of Stress
1. Director of Affairs. DOA's are continental directors for Campus Crusade for Christ.
2. Gary Collins, *You Can Profit From Stress* (Santa Ana, CA: Vision House, 1977), pp. 13,14
3. Proverbs 12:25 (TLB).
4. King James Version.
5. Bill and Deana Blackburn, *Stress Points in Marriage* (Waco, TX: Word Books, 1986), p. 17.
6. Robert A. Anderson, *Stress Power!* (New York: Human Sciences Press, 1978), p. 25.

### Chapter 3: The Stress of Sharing a Dream
1. Ephesians 5:22,23.
2. Genesis 2:24.
3. Ephesians 5:25.

### Chapter 4: The Stress of Role Confusion
1. Joyce Portner, *Stress and the Family* (New York: Brunner/Mazel Publishers, 1983), p. 164.
2. William Coleman, *Keeping Your Marriage From Burning Out* (San Bernardino, CA: Here's Life Publishers, 1989), p. 38.
3. Ephesians 5:22−6:4; 1 Corinthians 11:3 (TLB).

### Chapter 5: The Stress of Personality Differences
1. Romans 14:19 (NASB).
2. 1 Corinthians 13:7 (TEV).

### Chapter 6: The Stress of Being an Entrepreneur
1. Carla Wheeler, "Split Shift Couples," *The Sun* (October 1, 1989), p. E1.
2. John 15:12.
3. 1 John 5:14,15.
4. Matthew 25:14-30; Romans 14:12.

### Chapter 7: The Stress of Divided Loyalties
1. 1 Peter 5:7.
2. The Living Bible.

*Chapter 8: The Throne Check*

1. Ephesians 2:8.
2. Matthew 22:37,38 (NASB).
3. Psalm 1:1-3 (TLB).
4. John 15:7.
5. 1 Thessalonians 5:17.
6. 1 Peter 2:14-16 (NASB).
7. 1 John 1:9 (NKJV).
8. Ephesians 5:18.
9. 1 John 5:14,15.

*Chapter 9: Agree on Stewardship Principles*

1. Matthew 6:21.
2. Romans 1:1.
3. Galatians 6:7.
4. 1 Corinthians 16:2 (TLB).
5. Deuteronomy 14:23 (TLB).
6. Exodus 22:29,30.
7. 2 Timothy 2:4 (NASB).

*Chapter 10: The Power of Praise*

1. Romans 12:10 (TLB).
2. Ephesians 5:28,29 (RSV).
3. Ephesians 1:3.
4. Hebrews 13:15 (NKJV).
5. Leviticus 22:21.

*Chapter 11: Intimacy Through Communication*

1. 2 Timothy 1:7 (NKJV).
2. Psalm 34:13 (NASB).
3. Proverbs 15:4 (NASB).

*Chapter 12: Sex: God's Gift for Stress Relief*

1. Genesis 2:24.
2. Genesis 4:1.
3. 2 Corinthians 11:2 (NASB).
4. Ephesians 5:23,25,26,31,32 (TLB).

*Chapter 13: The Stress of Children*

1. Psalm 127:3-5 (TLB).
2. Proverbs 3:11,12.

*Chapter 14: Managing Family Crises*
1. James 1:2-4 (NIV).
2. Romans 8:29.
3. Psalm 37:4,5 (TLB).

*Chapter 16: Growing in Retirement*
1. Leviticus 19:32.
2. Proverbs 5:18 (TLB).
3. Job 5:26 (TLB).
4. Lee Gilliland, "Whitehead Talks, Africans Listen," *Worldwide Challenge* (February 1982), pp. 40-42.

*Chapter 17: Building a Home in a Pull-Apart World*
1. Proverbs 31:30 (TLB).
2. Proverbs 31:27 (TLB).
3. Proverbs 31:19,20 (TLB).
4. Proverbs 31:11.
5. Ephesians 5:22,23 (NIV).
6. Ephesians 5:21 (TLB).
7. 1 Peter 3:5.
8. Matthew 20:26-28 (NIV).
9. Proverbs 31:25 (TLB).
10. Proverbs 31:28,29 (TLB).

*Chapter 18: Radical Lover—Intimate Leader*
1. Ephesians 5:23 (NIV).
2. 1 John 4:19 (NIV).
3. Romans 5:6-8 (TLB).
4. 1 Peter 3:7 (NIV).
5. Philippians 2:5-8 (TLB).
6. Ephesians 5:23 (NIV).
7. Mark 16:15; Matthew 28:19.
8. Mark 10:43-45 (NIV).
9. Luke 22:25,26 (TLB).
10. John 13:6 (TLB).
11. John 13:4-9 (TLB).

# Bill Bright's Bestsellers

Quantity                                                                    Total

_____ **WITNESSING WITHOUT FEAR: How to Share Your**          $_____
**Faith With Confidence.** A warm, step-by-step approach to
overcoming common witnessing fears, sharing your faith with
loved ones, and the importance of prayer. Winner of the Gold
Medallion Award. ISBN 0-89840-176-3/$7.95

_____ **THE SECRET: How to Live With Purpose and Power.** An   $_____
intensely personal book, giving the reader a clear understanding of the ministry of the Holy Spirit in the life of the
believer. Filled with stories of people who have discovered the
dynamic of the Spirit-filled life. ISBN 0-89840-243-3/$7.95

_____ **PROMISES: A Daily Guide to Supernatural Living.** A    $_____
unique devotional which guides Christians to meditate and act
on one of God's promises each day. ISBN 0-86605-178-3/$9.95

_____ **AS YOU SOW: The Adventure of Giving by Faith.** A      $_____
refreshing biblical perspective enriched by stirring examples of
those who gave sacrificially and harvested deeper faith and joy.
ISBN 0-89840-262-X/$9.95

_____ **MANAGING STRESS IN MARRIAGE: Help for Couples**        $_____
**on the Fast Track.** Turn stressful moments into marriage en-
hancers! Bill and Vonette Bright share steps to make stress
work for you, to expand your personal effectiveness and grow
together as a couple. ISBN 0-89840-272-7/$7.95

**Order Total** $_____

---

Indicate product(s) desired above. Fill out below.
Send to:

**HERE'S LIFE PUBLISHERS, INC.**
P. O. Box 1576
San Bernardino, CA 92402-1576

NAME_____

ADDRESS_____

STATE_____ZIP_____

☐ Payment (check or money order only)
   included
☐ Visa    ☐ Mastercard #_____

Expiration Date_____Signature_____

**FOR FASTER SERVICE**
**CALL TOLL FREE:**
**1-800-950-4457**

| | |
|---|---|
| **ORDER TOTAL** | $_____ |
| SHIPPING and HANDLING | $_____ |
| ($1.50 for one book, $0.50 for each additional. Do not exceed $4.00.) | |
| APPLICABLE SALES TAX (CA, 6%) | $_____ |
| **TOTAL DUE** | $_____ |
| PAYABLE IN US FUNDS. (No cash orders accepted.) | |

MSM 272-7

Your Christian bookstore should have these in stock. If not, use this "Shop-by-Mail" form.
PLEASE ALLOW 2 TO 4 WEEKS FOR DELIVERY.
PRICES SUBJECT TO CHANGE WITHOUT NOTICE.

# BUILDING BETTER FAMILIES

## Practical Resources
## to Strengthen Your Home

Quantity                                                                    Total

____ **FAMILY FITNESS FUN** *by Charles Kuntzleman.*   $_____
Enjoy the sense of freedom that comes with feeling
healthier and more energetic by tapping into this
hassle-free handbook to a wholesome family lifestyle.
A book for the entire family with over 180 stimulating
strategies and activities for both parents and children.
ISBN 0-89840-279-4/$9.95

____ **HELPING YOUR KIDS HANDLE STRESS** *by H.*   $_____
*Norman Wright.* Whether your child is a toddler or
teen, the author offers practical ways to spot a stress
problem, identify its source, and help your child learn
to cope with stress successfully.
ISBN 0-89840-271-9/$7.95

____ **PULLING WEEDS, PLANTING SEEDS: Grow-**   $_____
**ing Character in Your Life and Family** *by Dennis*
*Rainey.* An inspiring collection of pointed reflections
on personal and family life with an abundance of practical insights for everyday living.
ISBN 0-89840-217-4/hardcover, $12.95

____ **MOM AND DAD DON'T LIVE TOGETHER**   $_____
**ANYMORE** *by Gary and Angela Hunt.* Help and encouragement for youth and their parents who are
working through this confusing time. If a divorce has
happened in your family, your kids need to know that
they are not alone—or wierd—and that there is hope
for their future. ISBN 0-89840-199-2/$5.95

____ **TALKING WITH YOUR KIDS ABOUT LOVE,**   $_____
**SEX AND DATING** *by Barry & Carol St. Clair.* The
topic which strikes fear in the heart of every parent!
Learn to resolve your fears and build an atmosphere
of love, trust and ongoing interaction with your kids
on these vital topics. ISBN 0-89840-241-7/$7.95

____ **THE DAD DIFFERENCE: Creating an Environ-**   $_____
**ment for Your Child's Sexual Wholeness** *by Josh*
*McDowell and Dr. Norm Wakefield.* Sets the stage for
fathering that will dramatically improve parent/teen
relationships and reduce teen sexual excesses. Practical examples of role modeling and father/children activities. ISBN 0-89840-252-2/$8.95

(Continued on next page.)

1158116

| Quantity | | Total |
|---|---|---|
| \_\_\_\_ | **DATING, LOVE, SEX GIFT SET,** *Josh McDowell, Series Editor*. Making the right decisions for a great relationship . . . Series includes **DATING: PICKING (AND BEING) A WINNER, LOVE: MAKING IT LAST,** and **SEX: DESIRING THE BEST.** ISBN 0-89840-235-2/$19.95 | $\_\_\_\_\_ |
| \_\_\_\_ | **PARENTING SOLO** *by Dr. Emil Authelet.* Take the fear—and some of the frustration—out of single parenting. Helpful ideas for laying a strong biblical foundation, understanding your need for healing, and overcoming barriers that keep you and your children from growing and enjoying a fulfilling life. ISBN 0-89840-197-6/$7.95 | $\_\_\_\_\_ |
| \_\_\_\_ | **IS THERE LIFE AFTER JOHNNY? Standing Strong Through Your Child's Rebellion** *by Joy P. Gage*. A bold, biblical and personal look at emotional healing for the grieving parent of a wayward child. ISBN 0-89840-255-7/$7.95 | $\_\_\_\_\_ |

**Order Total** $\_\_\_\_\_

---

Indicate product(s) desired above. Fill out below.
Send to:

**HERE'S LIFE PUBLISHERS, INC.**
P. O. Box 1576
San Bernardino, CA 92402-1576

NAME_____

ADDRESS_____

STATE_____ZIP_____

☐ Payment (check or money order only) included
☐ Visa   ☐ Mastercard #_____

Expiration Date_____Signature_____

**FOR FASTER SERVICE
CALL TOLL FREE:
1-800-950-4457**

**ORDER TOTAL** $_____

SHIPPING and
**HANDLING** $_____
($1.50 for one book,
$0.50 for each additional.
Do not exceed $4.00.)

**APPLICABLE
SALES TAX** (CA, 6%)$_____

**TOTAL DUE** $_____
PAYABLE IN US FUNDS.
(No cash orders accepted.)

MSM 272-7

Your Christian bookstore should have these in stock. If not, use this "Shop-by-Mail" form.
PLEASE ALLOW 2 TO 4 WEEKS FOR DELIVERY.
PRICES SUBJECT TO CHANGE WITHOUT NOTICE.